# STUDY LESS
## and still *blitz* your
# MEDICAL EXAMS

Kell Tremayne | Patsy Tremayne

*To our family and good friends*

Edited by Kath Walters.
Typset by Liz Seymour, Seymour Design.
Printed and bound by Ingram Sparks.

National Library of Australia Cataloguing-in-Publication entry

Title: Study Less and Still Blitz Your Medical Exams

Subtitle: You wouldn't use old technology on patients, so don't use outdated study methods on yourself

ISBN: 978-0-6485482-1-8 (paperback)
ISBN: 978-0-6485482-2-5 (eBook)

Subjects: Psychology, physiology, communication, performance, education, neuroscience

# TESTIMONIALS

"Oh, to have met Patsy before it all. Before university and GAMSAT and medical school. Before interning and basic training and Fellowship. Before ever studying for, or sitting, an exam.

"This book, a little bit of Patsy, contains the tools to make succeeding a little easier and failure more productive. I continue to employ these techniques daily to the amusement of colleagues and patients alike!"

**Dr Fred A English**
MB BCh BAO Hons. BSc. Hons. (Physiol.) Dip. (Health Sci.) FRCEM FACEM
Consultant Emergency Physician, Perth Children's Hospital, Western Australia
Country Health, and St John of God Health Care


"The words 'Don't Panic' should be inscribed in large friendly letters on the cover of Patsy's new book. Written in an engaging and warm style, this book is a reassuring and helpful guide for medical specialty trainees.

"I recommend Patsy's performance coaching to all my intensive care trainees after my experience of Patsy's coaching and it's wonderful that her evidence-based and practical approach to study is now available for all my junior staff and medical students to read.

"Patsy's advice to treat the exam as a challenge (rather than a looming threat) inspired me to change my mindset towards studying and approach the exam with a new perspective. I particularly enjoyed the advice to sing or dance to music to relieve stress and depression. Even long after my Fellowship exam has passed, I use this technique to change the mood in my household on difficult mornings."

**Dr Joanna Longley FCICM, FACRRM, FRACGP**
Staff Specialist, Hervey Bay Hospital, Qld

"Postgraduate medical exams are best tackled by likening yourself to an athlete – your brain being your strongest yet most flexible muscle. The muscle that will be worked beyond what you thought was possible.

"Patsy's second book (written with her son, Kell) is an extension of her initial delivery of an approach to study, but now explores why we are not alone in the experience of what is an all-consuming vortex of work and study. This book could be completed front to back, or as per the chapter that applies to you. It's conversational, yet impassioned prose is designed for easy reading, which is perfect for any time-poor student tackling adult learning alongside life itself."

**Dr Kristen Tuffin MBBS**
Advanced Trainee in Anaesthesia (ANZCA)
Victorian Regional Training Network
Ballarat Health/Austin Hospital
Heidelberg, Victoria

"I was four months pregnant with our third son when I failed the RACGP written exams on my first attempt. After extended maternity leave, and returning to work part-time, my confidence to attack them again was in the gutter. I felt like I never had enough time to study everything I needed to know, and I was struggling to enjoy time with my family. I was totally overwhelmed and didn't believe I could do it.

"A friend recommended Patsy, and it was without a doubt the saving grace. Honestly, I only studied the way Patsy advised me to study. I breathed the way she advised me to breathe. I slept. I spent time with the family. And I trusted the science and physiology behind everything she was recommending, everything that is recommended in this book. My memory improved, my exam technique improved, and my quality of life was miraculously steady. I passed each written exam on the second go, and then my clinical exam the first time. I will be forever thankful for navigating my path to Fellowship with Patsy and cannot thank her enough."

**Dr Anna Corbin**
BMedSci MBBS FRACGP
RAAF Base Williamtown, Health Centre

"Patsy taught me to work smarter, not harder. She restored my faith in my own ability to pass the Fellowship exam. I recommend her to all my registrar colleagues, whether they are struggling or not."

**Dr Jean O'Riordan**
MB BCh BAO FRACS (Urol)

"Patsy's earlier book *Ace Your Medical Exams* distilled her vast knowledge and experience, focussing on clinical examinations. This new book by Patsy and Kell is based on their vast experience and illustrated through case-based teaching, which always appeals to medicos. If our junior doctors (and senior medical students) read it carefully and implement the key strategies for success, then contentment and happiness will follow!"

**Professor John Watson AM**
BSc (Hons 1), MB, BS (Hons1), MD (Syd), DPhil (Oxon), FRACP, GAICD

"Patsy and Kell have a wealth of knowledge that they have taken the time to collate in this fabulous resource that I would strongly recommend to any doctor who is preparing for exams in their vocational training pathway. I was embarrassed to read through this book and reflect on how much well-meaning misdirection I have given to junior doctors in retelling war stories about my own marathon study timetable!

Instead, I will now be handing them a copy of this excellently constructed guide to much more efficient and effective study that will allow junior doctors to maintain their wellbeing and health while also achieving excellent academic results. Thank you both for supporting the medical profession in such a meaningful way."

**Dr Bronwyn Avard**
FCICM, MLMEd, PGCertCU, BMed
College Examiner

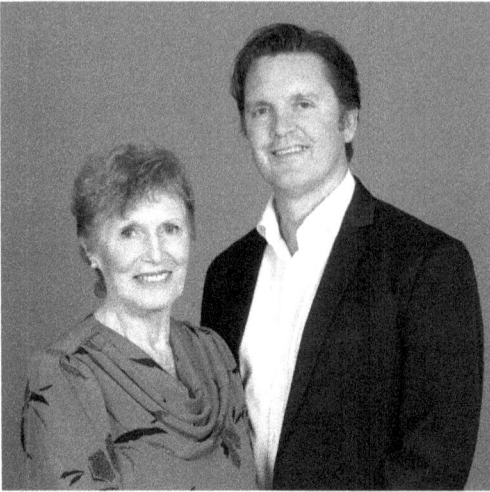

## ABOUT THE AUTHORS

Patsy and Kell have joined forces to combine their knowledge and experience in this book to help junior doctors ace their exams and triumph over a system that is stacked against them. This alliance has made for a very strong and dynamic psychology practice, with Patsy having decades of experience working in this industry, and Kell having an up-to-date rigorous research background.

Patsy and Kell have PhDs in psychophysiology and psychology respectively, and their career paths have many similarities.

For instance, both work at Western Sydney University. Patsy is an adjunct associate professor in psychology and Kell is a senior lecturer in the same department. At the same time, they each have different areas of expertise that they bring to this book. Kell lectures in subjects such as resilience, sleep hygiene, and factors that increase well-being and performance. Patsy loves non-verbal communication and the shortcuts to effective study and creative testing of exam components.

Kell and Patsy have had considerable experience working with elite athletes. Both have worked within the NSW Institute of Sport in areas that have involved wellbeing, management of stress and anxiety, and how to sustain motivation and confidence in the face of setbacks and challenges.

Patsy gives presentations to junior doctors around the country in many of the major specialties. Kell is in demand within the corporate world for his knowledge in elite performance in areas of leadership, time management, psychological safety, and stress management.

They would like nothing better than to see the long journey to finally becoming consultants in their chosen specialties be less fraught. It doesn't have to be that way, and in some small way, they hope this book can ease that transformation from junior doctor to a consultant.

# FOREWORD

Hundreds of doctors have sat in the clinic of Dr Patsy Tremayne in the months and weeks leading up to major examinations and bared their souls to her. Some come in, sure they know their key strengths and weaknesses, and others question their direction in medicine. Still, others have suffered from confidence or anxiety issues. I was one of those doctors and since then have sent countless trainees to her for guidance and careful counselling. For each of them, Patsy worked out a plan of action, unpacked the gravest of obstacles into smaller steps, and helped them face the demands of the job. She is, in short, a healer's healer.

This wonderful book places that knowledge into the hands of all clinicians. It concentrates on strategies and key examples that illuminate the pathway to success. Chapters on techniques include voice and non-verbal communication, appearance, and effective study. Patsy has gathered the evidence around maximising outcomes for the effort that is demanded of these clinicians when facing their final examinations in a chosen specialty.

Galen wrote in the 2nd century, "that physician will hardly be thought very careful of the health of others who neglects his own". Over the years, I have encountered a lot of unhappy but successful doctors. They get so busy giving to others that they forget to nurture their own souls and care for their own bodies. This book deals with wellbeing and mindfulness for clinicians. More importantly, it makes the point that mental wellbeing is as important as the physical and lays out careful strategies to guide the clinician.

Patsy has co-written this excellent text with her son, Kell, an eminent psychologist in his own right. Those of us who have relied on her wonderful guidance and extraordinary ability to bring out the best performance in us are celebrating Kell's engagement in this field and the continuation of this vital work.

I thoroughly recommend this book to all clinicians and not just to those who are facing the challenges of examinations and the tribulations of interviews.

**Professor Mohamed Khadra AO**
**B Med, Grad Dip Comp, MEd, PhD, FAICD, FRACS**
Professor of Surgery
Sydney Medical School
University of Sydney, NSW
Clinical Director of Surgery
Nepean Hospital, NSW

# CONTENTS

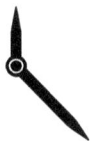

# INTRODUCTION

**I**s it really possible to study less and ace your exams? Absolutely. This probably flies in the face of all the advice you are given by your consultants. The received wisdom is that to prepare for your exams you need to be studying at every given opportunity. But is this the most effective way to learn? Absolutely not.

Science knows a lot more now about the brain and how it works. You don't need to put your life on hold until you pass those final exams. The trick is to study smarter, not longer. This book will show you how to optimise your study by using brain-based strategies that increase retention and recall. This is not easy as the study is more intense and more focused, but the content will stick, and you will still have time for other aspects of your life.

As soon as you open Chapter One, you will immediately see how life can change for you. You can not only improve your chances of acing your next round of medical exams, but life will be better, starting today.

This book will also bust some myths about resilience (it's not just about toughing it out), taking time out to socialise, exercise or do things that make you happy (it's not an indulgence you can't afford) and sleep (it's not taking time away from your study).

We will show you a range of techniques to improve your performance in exams, from better retention and recall to clearer communication and more confident presentation. These techniques are backed by science and proven to work. And importantly, they have helped hundreds of junior doctors who have come to us for help to pass their exams.

Most of our clients come to us because they are worried about upcoming exams. But what becomes clear is that these doctors seem to be at the end of their tether. They are exhausted. When questioned, many of them tell us that they are studying hard but can't remember the material a week later. Others have sleep issues – they toss and turn when they first go to bed, or they wake up in the early hours of the morning and can't get back to sleep. Many of them look pale and unfit. Does this sound familiar? Do you feel overwhelmed by the enormity of the task ahead of you, which you have to squeeze in around your already demanding workload as a doctor? Are you putting everything on hold, including looking after yourself, to focus on study?

Our approach to studying for your exams is a wholistic one. Your physical and emotional wellbeing are as important as your study. In fact, they are essential. Instead of being put on the back burner, you will discover that your wellbeing is the key to your success.

By prioritising your wellbeing, you increase your chances of exam success. Small differences make a big impact. You are in a demanding job, and if you can increase your wellbeing and resilience, you'll also reduce your chances of stress, anxiety, depression, and burnout, which unfortunately are all too common in your profession.

All junior doctors are up against a dysfunctional system. Burnout has reached epic levels. Burnout has been reported as high as 75% among Australian doctors, with the highest rates among junior doctors. Almost every doctor we speak to confirms this research, telling us they are burnt out, exhausted, and have no reserves.

We want to see the medical system become more compassionate towards young doctors. It doesn't need to be the gruelling journey that it was for previous generations of doctors. We want you to pass your exams. Then, later, down the track, you can use your influence to make lasting changes in the medical system.

But first, while you are still working and studying under this extreme duress, we can help you perform at your best with the time and energy you have.

## NOTE ON TERMINOLOGY

We work with both doctors-in-training on accredited programs in various specialties and junior doctors who are not on accredited training programs. For consistency, we are referring throughout the book to "junior doctors" or to "registrars".

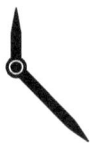

# CHAPTER ONE

# MORE ISN'T BETTER

Junior doctors are under the pump! It's a challenging environment in which you work. And then you're overwhelmed by the study as well. So, what will we discuss in this chapter? First, the mistaken belief that more study is better. Second, we'll show you that you can get side-tracked by what is going on around you no matter how well you plan. Third, often you're so exhausted with shift work and study, and life seems to be on hold, that there's no gas left in the tank. We'll discuss strategies to address that. Finally, a look at your previous experience of preparing for exams and see if that works for you now.

As you know, life as a junior doctor is busy, and it doesn't leave much time for anything else. The study tends to fit around work shifts, other activities, and chores. There's no set time, and some of you get told by consultants, *"You need to study every second of the day. Anytime you've got free time, you've got to study."* One junior doctor was told (facetiously but accurately) by her consultant, *"The primary exams are there to make you suffer. Then when you've suffered enough, they'll let you pass."* You've been told that lots of study is what is going to get you through, so you probably have the mistaken belief that more is better.

## MILLIE'S STORY, TOLD BY PATSY

*A dermatology registrar, Millie, came to see me. Millie was a conscientious and hard-working doctor who had been studying long hours, but not always effectively and efficiently. Over the six months prior to her several exams (all within a few weeks of each other), Millie became adept at studying less but retaining the material. She was using our techniques and was happy with the results from the first exams. But the closer she got to the last exam the more anxious she became. She kept thinking, "It's not enough. I've got to do more." She reverted to her old study habits and was studying in every spare moment. Millie was doing more than I had asked her to do. Finally, in her second to the last appointment before the exams, Millie broke down and said, through her tears, "Patsy, I can't do it anymore. I'm so anxious. This is no good. It's not working for me." When I asked her what she was doing, I was taken aback at how much more study and testing Millie was trying to fit in. This dermatology registrar had two young kids and was working night and day. She was seldom seeing her children.*

*I said, "Okay, that's it. You're going to do a lot less. You must focus on your wellbeing." Millie was so burnt out that she just did not argue. Instead, she took my advice. At her last appointment, about a week before the exam, she said, "I feel so much better. I feel fresher. I can do this now. I'm ready for this exam." During the last week, I instructed her to focus more on wellbeing, not cramming, and to do some meticulous planning for the day. Millie didn't know her results when we spoke, but she was pleased with how the exam day went. Weeks later, we found out that she had passed all her exams with merit.*

When doctors make an appointment to see us, they're often exhausted. They can't focus adequately on their studies. What they're learning isn't sticking, because a few weeks down the track, they can't remember important information when they get tested. If the consultant asks them a question, their minds just go blank. They're too tired to be motivated to study. So we're dealing with tired doctors who are studying excessively but ineffectively.

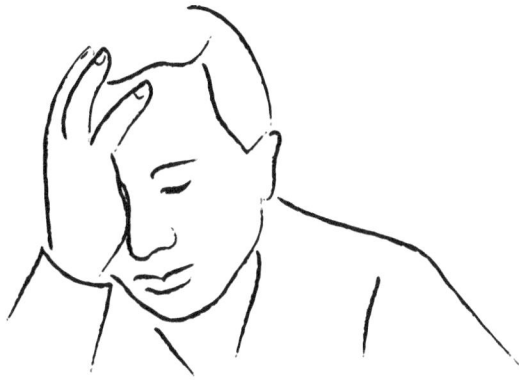

There are lots of unknowns. In some cases, these doctors are single, and you'd think they'd be all right. But what we find is that these junior doctors don't see their friends or have a social life. They're working long hours, shift work, and overtime. If they do socialise, it's with other healthcare workers because they work similarly unmanageable hours and understand. Other junior doctors have partners who work in unrelated fields, who have trouble understanding why they don't see much of each other. Again, other doctors have young children, toddlers, or babies while working these shift hours. They miss seeing their children. They don't see their friends very much either, or if they do, it's on the spur of the moment.

These doctors have difficulty committing to family celebrations or weddings unless they can get someone else to take their place on the roster. And most hospitals are understaffed these days.

As a result of all this these doctors are exhausted. The closer the exam comes, the more anxious, depressed, burnt out, and demotivated they feel.

Their number one failure seems to be planning. Rather than setting aside time for study, they try to study at every available moment.

> If you set time aside for specific study rather than studying whenever you can, you will feel better and be more in control.

## MORE STUDY IS NOT NECESSARILY BETTER

Junior doctors always think that more study is better because this is what they get told by consultants and what they see other trainees doing. For some consultants, it almost seems to be a badge of honour to tell junior doctors that they did lots of study when they were younger. But, like the pain of childbirth, these consultants have forgotten many of the details. They forget that doing this study takes away from the rest of your lifestyle. You put the rest of your life on hold, and you don't see your friends. You don't even realise that you are slowly deteriorating, physically and mentally, by constantly doing so much study. Think of that analogy of a frog sitting in warm water as it slowly comes to a boil.

But it doesn't have to be this way. You can still do well if you study smart, which means studying for specific study hours with short breaks. These short bursts of intense focus make the learning stick. By planning time for specific study, you can arrange to see friends. Your family knows when you're available and can work around that.

### CHRISTINE'S STORY, TOLD BY KELL

*After a year on maternity leave, Christine, a junior doctor, had been back at work a couple of months. Christine didn't realise what a struggle it would be, juggling full-time work, evening and night shifts, study, upcoming exams, and a young baby. She found that making time for study was always at the back of her mind. Her Fellowship exams were not too far away. Christine would be rocking the baby to sleep or perhaps taking time to play with her in the bath, and instead of mindfully enjoying the moment, she would have pangs of guilt at not being at her desk studying.*

*There's a saying, "I've got a monkey on my back." And this is the way Christine felt. She couldn't enjoy any free moments away from her desk because of that so-called monkey. It kept reminding her that she ought to be doing more study. It was getting her down. So, she came to me to get some professional time-management advice.*

*Christine seemed to be so much happier towards the end of her first session. I was able to organise and suggest specific times on her days off to study. These hours were the same, whatever days she had off, and it enabled her and her partner to organise their shopping and see friends outside those study times. This meant that she was able to be more mindful when playing with the baby or doing other activities and studying didn't impinge too much on other aspects of her life. She said, with a big sigh of relief, "It's so good to have a plan." It was as though a weight had been lifted from her shoulders.*

*Christine emailed me a few weeks later. She felt so much better. The new study plan had given her confidence, and she felt she was learning and retaining the material.*

Are you of the opinion that you need to study every waking moment? Do you get study advice from respected fellows and consultants? Are you told that the only way to get through these exams is to just put your head down, put everything on hold, and study as hard as you can? Do you get assured that it worked for them?

## What you can do right now to make a change

This is just for fun! Make a note or give a score out of 10 on how often you're told by consultants, supervisors, or other trainees that you need to study in almost every free moment. Do they suggest you study every night after work? Or perhaps they say that you should start in the morning and work until dusk on every day off. Do they tell you how they passed because they followed that advice? Has that advice motivated you or disheartened you? When you note down how often you get that advice, especially from your seniors, it's hard to believe that there can be another way.

The benefit of doing this exercise is that you realise you should stick to scientific principles. It's going to be less confusing!

## YOU CAN GET SIDE-TRACKED

There are several stumbling blocks, such as family emergencies and illnesses, which can side-track a junior doctor when preparing for exams. The big one is, of course, the pandemic.

Many changes have had to take place. COVID has affected all the colleges. Out of necessity, there were alterations in exam schedules. Some exams were postponed, and some were cancelled. Exams that entailed examiners visiting from interstate had to be altered so that only local examiners were used for face-to-face encounters. In many instances, real patients are no longer used. Many exams were conducted on virtual platforms, such as Zoom, and still are being conducted that way. They may never go back to the old normal. And it looks as though there will be a new normal for the structure of exams in some specialties.

Quite apart from the exams, the pandemic affected the training schedule of many doctors. Some of you were not trained in your specialties, and hospitals were stretched to the limit. Many of you were deployed to frontline tasks, and elective surgery was cancelled or reduced during the crisis. It made a big difference to the mental health of all healthcare staff who went through this crisis.

As doctors, you are on the front lines of the continuing COVID fight. Unfortunately, it looks as though this fight will be around for some time, in some form or other, until most people on the planet have been vaccinated and there is more freedom of movement.

There is the pressure of constantly dealing with COVID, and it has changed how you manage infection control at the hospital, in the clinic, at home, and out in society. There is mental wear and tear, emotional toll, and long-term impact. Given the magnitude and the fact that this pandemic continues with different variants, the major consequences are psychological. There is fear, and there is economic and social dislocation. There are mental health risks, especially as you read about what has been happening overseas and know it is happening here. Being on edge all the time is emotionally exhausting.

Doctors are generally organised, disciplined, and motivated people. However, uncertainty is always unsettling. There's emotional distress, and your worried mind can be burdened with distractions. The uncertainty of this virus has meant that doctors have had to exercise an unprecedented level of caution to protect their patients, themselves, and their family from infection when they go home at night. Constant hypervigilance drains energy.

All medical colleges have had to change how they do their written and oral examinations, and this has caused slip-ups and disruptions. It's hard to focus and be motivated to prepare for exams under these abnormal conditions.

Fairly early in the pandemic, Patsy recalls working with a senior registrar from Sydney called Alex, who had planned to be sitting his Fellowship exam in August 2020.

Alex and his wife, Sacha, also a doctor, had planned their first pregnancy well. The baby was due in September, a month after completing his exam. His wife's parents were planning to fly up from Melbourne to assist with the baby while Sacha prepared for her exam the following February. Patsy was very impressed with all the planning that had taken place. It was all organised very well. But, of course, no one could foresee the disruptions that were to take place during that year.

Alex's exam was postponed because of COVID, and the college advised that the exam would be held in October 2020. The baby was born in September, one month before Alex's exams. There was considerable disruption with a new baby in the home, and the plan to have the grandparents there to assist went out the window. They were in lockdown in Melbourne and were unable to help.

Sadly, Alex failed this exam due partly to sleepless nights with a newborn baby. He ended up doing the exam a few months later and was relieved to pass at his second attempt, but Sacha decided to postpone her exam until a few months later.

It all worked out in the end, but I think this is a particularly good example of how junior doctors can get side-tracked from their study and exam goals, even after meticulous planning.

## What you can do right now to make a change

### INCREASE YOUR AWARENESS BY TRACKING YOUR INTERRUPTIONS

Make a note of how often you're interrupted, distracted, or lose track of what you're doing. Then note how many times you're so side-tracked that you don't do what you plan to do that day, week, or month.

The benefits of noting this down are that you develop more awareness. Later in the book, we'll show you how to overcome being side-tracked.

## NO GAS LEFT IN THE TANK

Junior doctors like you are so tired and burnt out that you often don't have the energy to see friends or have much of a social life. It's sometimes easier to hang out with other healthcare workers who understand the problems of working irregularly on the day, evening, or night shifts. We notice that you often cut down on your daily exercise, perhaps because it takes you away from studying, or maybe shift work prevents you from attending your favourite exercise classes. The associated increase in burnout due to shift work, overtime, and study often leads to increased negative emotion. Examples are a loss of motivation and a sense of failure, incompetence, and self-doubt, especially around the study. Overall, you develop an increasingly cynical and negative outlook. The fear that you feel around exams is heightened.

Deterioration of physical or mental health over the weeks and months starts to affect your ability to integrate study material into long-term memory. Often you can't focus your attention appropriately when you do study, which increases your stress, your sabotaging thoughts, your procrastination, and the feeling that you're out of control.

## EDDIE'S STORY, TOLD BY PATSY

*One young doctor, Eddie, came to see us because he just couldn't see any way forward. He had failed his Fellowship written exam twice. He now had a mental health plan and had started seeing a psychologist for depression and anxiety.*

*Eddie was one of those doctors who believed that he had to study whenever there was spare time. His second failure at the written exam upset him. He was ashamed and felt that he had let his family down. He also described how embarrassed he was to go to work the day after getting his exam results. Many of his colleagues from the same year in med school were now fellows or junior consultants. Eddie was starting to wonder if he was competent enough to continue.*

*When I questioned him closely, it seemed apparent that little information was being absorbed during Eddie's study times. Eddie was too exhausted because he was always studying after work and spent most of his days off at his desk. He didn't have a girlfriend anymore and wasn't seeing much of other friends. He complained that he had gained weight because he had stopped doing regular exercise a few months back.*

*After a little more fact-finding, I gave Eddie a specific study plan, which was quite a few hours less than he had previously allocated for study. I felt that Eddie was probably bored with going over the curriculum in the same way. He could do less study, but with much more focus on maintaining his attention to the task. So, I asked him to study in the morning of his days off, change topics regularly, and start with a topic he disliked. And he was to take a 10-minute break every 50 minutes.*

*Eddie was dubious about studying shorter hours. But his eyes lit up when he realised that he was free to see friends and get some exercise on the afternoons of his days off work. I asked Eddie to give feedback after two or three weeks of this new study plan. He discovered that he liked it. He found that working for short periods and then having a quick break improved his mood, and he felt more in control. He also told me that what he learned seemed to be sticking.*

This is an example of a junior doctor who was suffering a deterioration in his mental and physical health. However, with more focus on wellbeing and time allocated to exercising, socialising, and generally getting a life, Eddie overcame burnout and successfully continued his medical training.

## What you can do right now to make a change

### MONITOR YOUR MOOD

Make up your own anxiety exercise. Rank yourself out of 10 when you awaken and again on retiring. A score of 10 could be that you feel depressed and anxious, whereas a score of one or two could be that you feel positive, even excited.

It's quite likely that in the morning, after a good night's sleep, you feel positive and energetic. However, as you move through the day and realise you're not getting through all the tasks you had planned to do, you become more and more depressed. You end up giving yourself a high score by the time you go to bed. Next to the score, just write a reflective sentence about why you feel that way.

After a week or two, look back on these scores and comments and see how you're coping.

The benefit of doing this exercise is that you become aware of the need to be more realistic about what can be achieved each day. And that it's worth it to plan short recovery breaks.

## YOUR PREVIOUS EXPERIENCE OF EXAMS WORKS AGAINST YOU

To get accepted into med school, you must be bright. You probably did exceptionally well in your final school exams, and you were near the top of your class. When you were younger, you could study at night efficiently, and the material would stick. Most of you made it into med school in your early twenties. Cramming was common. You were able to study at night and could stay up late. Exams at university covered just that semester's work, which is typical for most university students. And usually, the exams consisted of multiple-choice questions. But this changes for doctors when they sit their exams many years later before becoming consultants.

The exams you must study for now consist of the whole curriculum in your specialty. And you may have a variety of written and oral exam components – not just multiple-choice questions. You can't cram that sort of thing. You also now have a mature brain; you're probably in your thirties by this time and studying in the morning is more effective. The amount of information that can potentially be tested is so enormous that you need to ascertain which topics have the most value in exams. And now, all the study needs to be fitted around a full-time job and a family.

### AHMED'S STORY, TOLD BY KELL

*Ahmed was an anaesthetic registrar. He worked a minimum of 12 hours a day. He came home from work, and he studied until bedtime. He studied most of the day with small breaks on his days off. He was exhausted. When questioned by consultants, he didn't seem to remember any of the material he had studied. This was getting him down. Having been a top student in med school and his school life, he now felt incompetent. He was embarrassed. He'd already failed once, and he was devastated. His techniques weren't working for this major exam, which covered the whole curriculum.*

*I suggested that Ahmed set aside an hour every night to test exam components. He was to set aside just the mornings for study on his days off, with short breaks for recovery each hour. And in the afternoons on his days off, he was to "get a life" – in other words, focus more on wellbeing, and spend time with friends and family.*

*I gave him the analogy of a sculptor with a big lump of clay to make a statue. The statue can't be sculpted overnight or even in a few days; instead, the sculptor must chip away, steadily and consistently over many months. It's the same with study and testing for specialist exams – progress may seem slow, especially at the beginning, but little by little, with constant effort, you can achieve your goal. This analogy resonated with Ahmed. He wasn't sitting again for a few months, so he had time to adjust to his new study schedule. He found that his understanding of material improved, his confidence returned, and he passed at his second attempt.*

We know it's challenging to study with shift work, lack of exercise, juggling family and social life, and all the other sorts of activities in your life. This is another reason why trying to cram for your exam as you did in high school is not a practical option.

> There is no need to spend your whole evening with your books. Set aside an hour each night to do specific testing of exam components.

Note any errors you have made as soon as you have finished the testing but don't try to read around the topic then. Wait for a morning study session when your brain is fresh.

## SUMMARY

If you have been making the number one mistake most junior doctors make, which is to believe that you must study at every opportunity, then you can now take that pressure off yourself. Now you know that you can study smarter, with fewer hours, and still ace your exams.

We've had emails from junior doctors saying, *"I'm keeping focused and finding the tools we discussed very helpful."* or *"Practising in this way is already enough to boost up my morale."* Another one – *"Thank you so much for your words of wisdom and for helping me prepare a game plan. It made such a difference! And I will be taking the lessons learned forward."* Many doctors just remark at the end of the first session and say, *"I'm so relieved I now have a study plan."*

In the next chapter, we demonstrate how you can have more time with friends and family, get some exercise, have some fun, and still get through those upcoming exams. Wouldn't it be great to feel normal again?

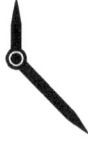

# CHAPTER TWO

# WELLBEING AND SUCCESS MAKE A GREAT TEAM

The World Health Organization (WHO) defines health as a *"state of complete physical, mental, and social wellbeing and not merely the absence of disease or infirmity."* This definition implies that a healthy body fuelled with a nourishing diet, and exercise, and healthy social relationships are crucial for a healthy mind. This chapter shows how wellbeing improves your brain function. It highlights that focusing on your wellbeing does not come at a net cost to your study time. Wellbeing is not a luxury; it's necessary for optimal brain performance. When you focus on your wellbeing, you optimise your brain. As a result, you give yourself the best opportunity to pass your exams.

For most doctors we talk with, when there is an upcoming important exam, almost everything gets pushed to the side to focus on their studies. Unfortunately, this can mean that other aspects of their lives are put on hold. This includes relationships with loved ones, health, exercise, spending time with friends, or pursuing hobbies – the very things that support their wellbeing and resilience. The removal of these supports:

- diminishes the doctor's quality of life
- increases their vulnerability to increased stress and burnout
- reduces the chances of optimising their brain to pass their exams.

Consider a Formula 1 car, a very complex machine that travels upwards of 320 kilometres an hour. The pit stop is crucial to the car's performance during the race. Without a pit stop, it would be challenging to complete the entire race due to the wear and tear on the vehicle. In the pit stop, the car will pause to change tyres, refuel, and make mechanical adjustments. Each of these factors is critically important to the speed and performance of the Formula 1 car. Efficiency at the pit stop can mean the difference between winning and losing the race.

> The pit stop is a metaphor for deliberate recovery and rejuvenation that you need to take both within your study and in your days.

Studying efficiently and effectively relies on optimal brain performance. Do not underestimate the importance of exercise, sleep, and managing stress. Getting these things right provides a platform for quality study and optimal retention.

## MOTION IS MEDICINE

Imagine if you could take a pill that could make you lose weight, look younger, improve your sleep, and help you to reduce stress. What if this pill could also optimise your brain and, therefore, your chances of getting through your exam? If we were to tell you that this pill is freely available, every newspaper would headline this information. The magic pill is exercise.

Of course, you are familiar with the benefits of regular physical activity on wellbeing and the corresponding cardiovascular and respiratory benefits. But did you know that physical activity improves learning and memory? In his book *Spark*, Dr John J Ratey, a clinical professor of psychiatry at Harvard Medical School, tells us that exercise improves learning on three levels:

1. Exercise helps balance neurotransmitters critical for learning, attention, and focus.
2. Physical activity facilitates the birth and growth of new nerve cells from stem cells in the hippocampus.
3. Exercise helps to encourage nerve cells to bind to one another, which means that exercise helps memory stick.

So, the direct benefits of exercise are that it primes your brain to learn and allows your brain to retain information easier.

Dr Ratey's research also points to several other indirect benefits of exercise: physical activity improves mood, increases sleep, and counters the effects of chronic stress.

Our clients often say that exercise is a luxury they can't afford. While they know that exercise helps them get healthy or improve their mood – they can't afford the time away from their study.

Dr John Ratey's research shows that you
can view exercise with a different lens – a lens in
which exercise is not seen as time away from study
but as something that enhances the quality
and retention of the study.

Suddenly, exercise is not just a vehicle to stay fit or improve your mood but is essential to enhance your thinking and study quality.

Several studies have shown that regular exercise improves the learning and memory of young adults. However, we particularly like Peter Blomstrand and Jan Engvall's meta-analysis of 13 studies published in *Translational Sports Medicine*. This study looked at the effects of a single bout of moderate to high-intensity exercise (walking, running, and bicycling) that lasted between two minutes and one hour. They found that a single episode of physical activity before the study increased the encoding, consolidation, and retrieval of content that was studied over the next two hours. In other words, they learned the content better, with the researchers remarking that *"exercise makes you smart"*.

## KATE'S STORY, TOLD BY PATSY

*Kate was a young doctor who put everything aside to focus on her exam. "This exam has caused so much distress over the last two years. I've put everything aside so I can study. I find I'm crying every day over almost nothing. If I stop and do nothing, all my negative thoughts overwhelm me. So, I keep going. I just study whenever I can find a spare moment. I'm missing out on my kids, I'm not getting any real exercise, and I know my mental health is deteriorating. I used to enjoy going to aerobic classes down at the gym. I just can't find the time now. Medicine is not giving me much joy anymore."*

*After talking with Kate for a while, it was clear that she needed to make some changes. She had already failed the exam once, and if she continued in the same way, there was a good chance she would fail again. We agreed that it was probably too challenging to get to a regular aerobics class. Kate had a roster that included evening and night shifts. However, we talked about the benefits of high-intensity interval training. This could be done every day, or every second day, it didn't take up too much time, and it could be done at home. Kate read up on it and then booked a personal trainer for a couple of sessions. This personal trainer organised a weekly program that Kate could do herself. It was flexible and suited Kate's schedule.*

*After a few weeks, the change in Kate's demeanour was noticeable. She smiled a lot more, had lost some weight, and was more optimistic. She set aside specific times for study. By doing this, Kate felt she had more control over her life. She wasn't trying to study at every moment. She didn't feel guilty when she made time to spend with her children. And the children benefited. They knew when Mum was studying and when she was available to be with them.*

In our experience, it can be challenging for time-poor junior doctors to get into a regular exercise routine. If you can do this, you will reap the benefits of exercise on your brain and subsequent learning. However, if a regular exercise routine remains aspirational for you, you can do small things that benefit your study and subsequent retention. For example, before sitting and studying, do some moderate to intense exercise for a few minutes (note that this can be as little as two minutes). Based on the above study, this will help to improve the encoding, consolidation, and retrieval of information for your subsequent study session.

## THE BEST WAY TO LEARN IS TO SLEEP ON IT

Compared to humans, giraffes sleep a relatively meagre two hours a day and koalas an indulgent 22 hours a day. But, irrespective of the differences in sleep hours, all animals give over a portion of their day to not chase, drink, eat, or guard themselves – and in this time, they sleep. So clearly, sleep is essential. You only need to miss a night's sleep to understand that sleep is crucial for wellbeing and how you feel on the job the next day.

But did you know that sleep is crucial for memory? And this is essential for learning. There are three broad processes to memory:

1. encoding the information coming in
2. consolidating or storing the encoded information in memory
3. retrieval of this information later.

The encoding and retrieval primarily occur during wakefulness, with much of the memory consolidation occurring during sleep.

Throughout the day, we form memories that can be fragile and delicate. While asleep, the brain sifts through the short-term memories, deciding what to keep and not to keep. There are likely two effects of this. The first is that sleep memory consolidation involves strengthening neural connections that form memories. As such, doctors are more likely to recall their studies later if they have had a good night's sleep. The second is that sleep helps sort the non-useful short-term memories that are subsequently forgotten. This "taking out the garbage" is essential for collecting more short-term memories and promotes efficient learning.

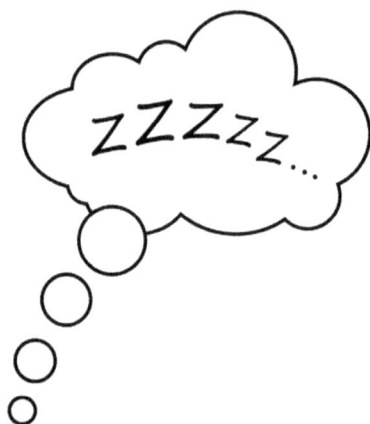

Often, doctors believe that sleep takes away from study. However, this is a mistaken belief. On the contrary, sleep is essential for quality study and retention of information.

## WHAT'S THE EVIDENCE?

In Australia, you're not fit to drive if you're over 0.05 in terms of your blood alcohol limit. Studies show that sleep deprivation, where someone is awake for 18 hours, is the equivalent of having a blood alcohol concentration of 0.05. Being awake for at least 24 hours pushes this up to the equivalent of 0.10 blood alcohol content. Some doctors do shifts longer than 24 hours, which means they're working on patients and saving lives under the same conditions that they would not legally be able to drive a car.

In our experience working with junior doctors, there is much uncertainty around your rosters.

> However, you can still optimise your sleep if you're building good sleep hygiene or recognising what you can do and what you shouldn't do when on night shifts.

You are probably already sleep-deprived, and you know full well how much of a wreck you are emotionally compared to if you've had a good night's sleep. However, do you practise good sleep hygiene?

## DAVID'S STORY, TOLD BY KELL

*David was in the theatre every day at 7.30 am. He would get home again anywhere between 7 and 9 pm. He would study until 1 am, and then try to sleep. David said he tossed and turned, had trouble getting to sleep, and was lucky to get three hours of sleep a night. He was constantly tired and wasn't remembering the material he read at night.*

*When I questioned him more closely, I discovered that David frittered away the time when he first came home. He sat on his phone looking at*

*Facebook while eating takeaway fried food. Then at about 11 pm, he tried to study till bedtime.*

*With a bit of coaxing, I managed to persuade David to change some of his night-time habits. He switched to more nutritious meals that would digest more easily overnight, which he prepared and froze a week in advance. On some days, he was able to eat before he left the hospital. He endeavoured to study when he first came home, rather than starting at 11 pm. He was in bed by midnight, and in the hour beforehand, he would relax and have some quiet time. If David wanted to use Facebook, he would use a device that did not rob the body of melatonin because of the blue light.*

*After a few weeks, David noticed the difference. He was more likely to get to sleep without tossing and turning. He digested his dinner before going to bed. And although he was still a bit sleep-deprived, he was getting around six hours of sleep a night. More importantly, David reported that he seemed to be remembering previously studied material a little better.*

## STRESS AFFECTS YOUR MEMORY

Stress is not all bad. We need stress to get up in the morning, and we need a little stress to be motivated and to hit deadlines. From an evolutionary point of view, the stress response serves an adaptive function to escape the sabre tooth tiger and live another day. However, today's figurative sabre tooth tiger – work deadlines, traffic, relationship problems, or worrying thoughts – mean that the stress response is always switched on. The sustained activation of the sympathetic nervous system (the stress response) involves a constant production of stress hormones.

The health impacts of chronic stress are many, including hypertension, fatigue, and depression, to name a few – all of which can affect your study and retention. However, chronic stress also has an impact on memory and learning.

In our practice, we often see junior doctors who have very high workloads, demanding work conditions, and continually try to balance work, study, and other obligations. Their high levels of chronic stress are likely a significant reason for the high burnout in the profession.

These high levels of chronic stress are likely to impair learning. Stress thwarts the development of short-term memories and the encoding of short-term memories into longer-term memories.

Stress can also impact the retrieval of memories. For example, you might notice this when you have practised and presented a perfect presentation to yourself in front of the mirror. But you find that your mind goes blank in front of an audience the following day!

A way to counteract the stress of your demanding job and packed schedule is to find time throughout the day to decompress and activate the parasympathetic nervous system. Activating the parasympathetic nervous system puts our body into a state of relaxation and recovery.

There are many ways to activate the parasympathetic nervous system, ranging from meditation and yoga to exercise and nutrition. While these are likely to be helpful, they can be challenging to incorporate into a hospital setting. In a hospital environment with limited spare capacity, breathwork is the easiest way for you to activate the parasympathetic nervous system.

Breathwork intentionally slows down
the breathing rate and lets your body
know everything is OK.

## What you can do right now to make a change

TRY THIS BREATHING EXERCISE

The following breathing exercise will activate the parasympathetic nervous system.

First, regularly practise inhaling for a count of four and exhaling for a count of four. Repeat this for up to ten breaths. Then, over a few weeks, look to increase the count to six to deepen the practice.

The benefits are that it's effective at calming yourself down and you can choose whenever and wherever you want to do it.

## SUMMARY

Wellbeing is not just reducing the waistline, looking younger, or feeling better – wellbeing also primes your mind for memory and learning. The core physical foundations of wellbeing don't occur in isolation. Each foundational habit supports and enriches the others. If you have a good night's sleep, you're better able to manage your stress. A good night's sleep gives you enough energy to contemplate morning exercise. Similarly, if you've done some exercise, you're more likely to eat healthily or manage your stress better.

These foundational habits are the fertile soil
in which your study habit will flourish as they will
improve your memory and concentration, allowing
you to study more efficiently and effectively.

Making positive changes, no matter how small, can have a significant impact. They improve the quality of how you feel and the quality of your thinking. You're more likely to get through those critical exams.

We've talked about some of the physical foundations of wellbeing and their positive impact on memory and learning. In the next chapter, we look at how we can build resilience and protect ourselves from burnout.

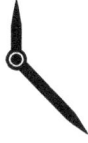

# CHAPTER THREE

# FROM BURNOUT TO RESILIENCE

There is a high level of burnout among Australian junior doctors. A contributing factor to burnout is stress, in particular chronic levels of stress. Managing your stress is about increasing your awareness of what causes your stress and how you typically respond to it. In this chapter, we discuss the common cognitive traps that reduce resilience, mindfulness-based techniques that help reduce stress, and how social or environmental factors can increase resilience.

Being a doctor can be an enriching and purposeful career. However, as you probably know, the incredibly demanding schedules, nights on call, and staying on top of your study and medical knowledge can make it very hard to balance competing work and personal demands. Even though doctors are a very resilient cohort, they suffer from significantly higher psychological distress and burnout levels than the general Australian population and other Australian professionals, according to the *National Mental Health Survey of Doctors and Medical Students*.

The transition from study to work (or studying while working) is a particularly stressful period for junior doctors. As a result, younger doctors are more vulnerable to poor mental health, higher levels of distress, and burnout than older doctors.

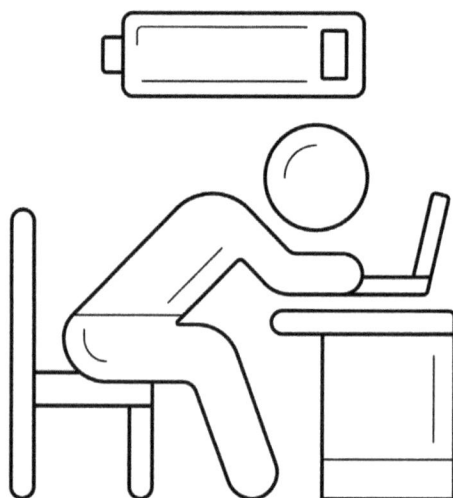

We're going to tackle some sensitive topics in this chapter, including a discussion of suicide. It is vital to get honest about this because so much is swept under the carpet. If this triggers any concerns for you, please call a support service:

- Lifeline –13 11 14
- Beyond Blue – 1300 22 4636

Burnout is defined by the experience of emotional exhaustion, depersonalisation, and reduced personal accomplishment. Burnout has reached epidemic levels among doctors with global prevalence rates of clinician burnout ranging from 25–75%, and Australian levels ranging from 65–75% according to the Australian Medical Association's position statement on the *Health and Wellbeing of Doctors and Medical Students.*

Burnout has a serious impact on productivity and wellbeing. Burnout leads to increased medical errors, reduced work hours, and increased suicidal ideation; therefore, we all have a vested interest in preventing burnout. To care for patients, doctors must maintain their health and wellbeing; and one avenue is to enhance resilience.

Resilience is typically defined as the capacity to recover from a challenging event. This does not mean that a resilient person doesn't have periods of stress, emotional upheaval, or pain; however, resilient people utilise their strengths and reach out to others to overcome challenges and setbacks. Resilience is not a fixed trait. Instead, it is a learnable skill. We'll be covering formal and informal strategies that you can put into practice to increase real-time resilience and reduce your chances of burnout.

Australian doctors have higher levels of stress and attempts at suicide than the general Australian population, according to the *National Mental Health Survey of Doctors and Medical Students*. According to Beyond Blue, there's an increased risk for junior doctors in their early stages of training. This is heartbreaking and likely to be much smaller than the actual number, which often doesn't make the newspapers or the statistics. So many of our clients come into the office, or meet with us on Skype or Zoom, and quickly break down in tears.

In our practice, we worked with a junior doctor who was told by one of her consultants that if you haven't cried on your first night shift, it's a good night shift. This assertion is not only untrue but also an unhelpful belief. This belief implies that, in the face of unrelenting stress, they should get on with it or that these bad experiences can be worn as a badge of honour – *"Hey, look what I can cope with."*

Unfortunately, dysfunctional coping strategies such as blame, self-distraction, and substance abuse can be common coping mechanisms and are not particularly helpful in the short or long term. We can see this in the high burnout figures among doctors and junior doctors.

## THE RELATIONSHIP BETWEEN STRESS AND BURNOUT

Burnout and stress are not the same things. However, increasing your resilience can help to reduce the chances of chronic stress and burnout. There are many reasons why doctors might reach the burnout stage. These include:

- a lack of control
- unclear job expectations
- dysfunctional work dynamics
- lack of social support
- struggling to balance work with other responsibilities.

According to Daniel Tawfik and colleagues' article published in the *Current Treatment Options in Pediatrics (2019)*, there's plenty of research showing that organisational factors, policies, and culture influence burnout rates in doctors and physicians. We agree – the system lets doctors down. That said, if you haven't got time to change the world, we want to give you strategies to cope at a personal level.

Resilience is not an immutable skill that you bring into the world with you. It's something that you can grow and maintain. If you can build or maintain your already high levels of resilience, you're better able to manage the challenges that work and life are likely to throw at you. According to the American Medical Association, resilience gives you skills to reduce your chance of burnout, help you be a better doctor, and pass your upcoming exams.

The doctors we meet are under unrelenting stress, and often they see resilience as making them tougher. But this is not true.

Resilience is about helping see the stressors in your world and responding to those stressors with a minimal psychological or physical cost.

As we mentioned in the last chapter, stress is not necessarily a bad thing. We need it to wake up in the morning, focus, learn, and remember new things. The fight or flight response evolved to help us escape from predators, so it also has an adaptive response. While there are not many wild animals in our environment now, the same stress response can get turned on when we are overwhelmed with work, stuck in traffic, or dealing with a difficult patient. When in a prolonged state, these stress responses can become chronic stress and lead to burnout. That's not much fun!

When stressed, you move through three phases in what's called the stress response.

1. the alarm phase – a fight or flight response
2. the resistance phase
3. the exhaustion stage.

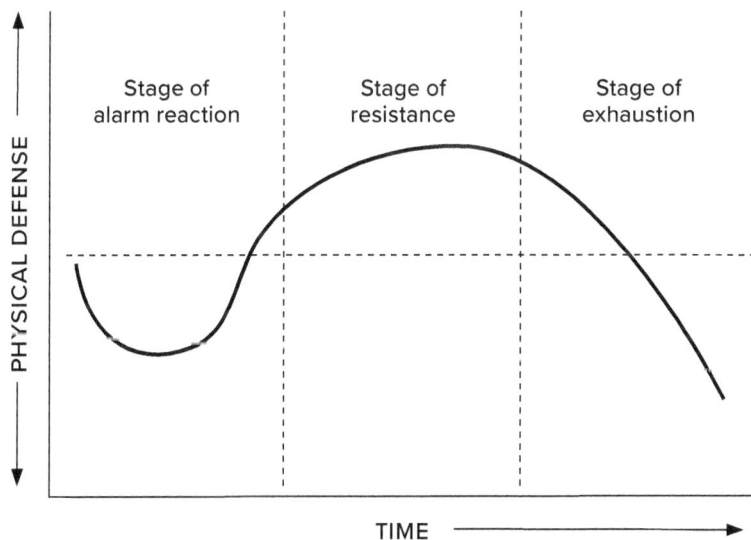

The exhaustion stage is characterised by increased burnout, depression, anxiety, and an inability to cope. Therefore, it's essential to have strategies to deal with unrelenting stress to minimise your time in the exhaustion phase of the stress response.

The bucket analogy for stress is widely used to help you visualise the idea of chronic stressors in your life, which might also lead to burnout. The size of the bucket – your stress tolerance – is the product of your genes, personality, and life experiences, so one person's stress bucket will be different from another's. The water in the bucket is all the stress in your life.

When you're confronted with stress like working beyond your competency levels, inadequate supervision or support, unrealistically high expectations of yourself, big workloads, pressure to sit exams, or relationship issues, this can be like rain that fills your stress bucket. While there are likely to be structural and organisational factors that can reduce the water coming into the bucket, there are also several things that you can do to reduce the water coming in, or to let it drain out. This might involve learning and finding new coping strategies and using several coping strategies.

Some of these self-care strategies could be:

- meditation
- self-awareness and self-regulation
- critical thought and analysis
- exercise
- quality of sleep
- relaxation
- sharing feelings with your friends or partner.

These self-care strategies can include problem-focused coping, which involves taking action to resolve the underlying cause of stress. In contrast, emotionally focused coping strategies involve regulating your feelings and response to the issue. Depending on the situation, both problem and emotionally focussed coping strategies can be helpful or unhelpful. For example, several unhelpful coping strategies might include staying up late, using drugs, inactivity, procrastination, ignoring or suppressing your feelings. In the stress bucket analogy, these are like false taps that might provide temporary relief but result in water flowing back into your bucket.

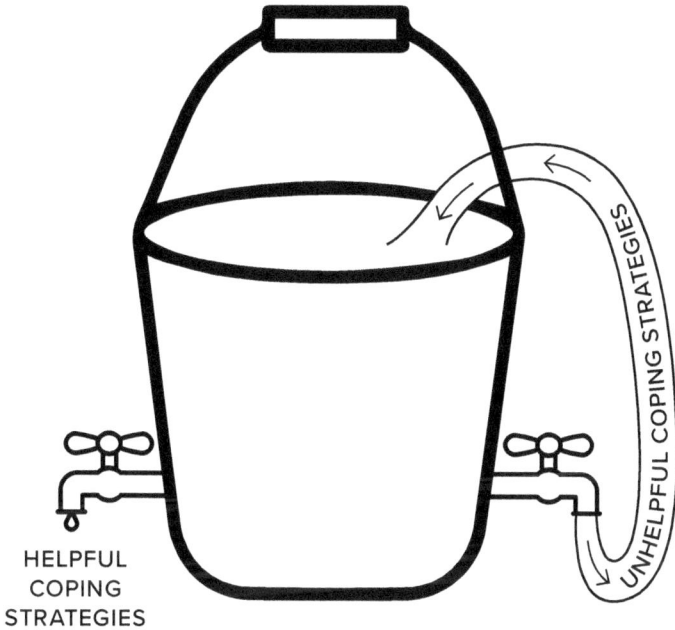

HELPFUL
COPING
STRATEGIES

UNHELPFUL COPING STRATEGIES

Years ago, Patsy remembers a surgical trainee who was bullied relentlessly by one consultant. Amy was exhausted and angry. This consultant made a point of questioning Amy even when she was operating in theatre. Although Patsy didn't know it at the time, Amy was increasing her alcohol use from just her day off each week, to after every shift. However, Patsy did notice that Amy was forgetful about appointments, and she was somewhat concerned that Amy was becoming depressed and more exhausted as the weeks went by. On the last occasion that Patsy had a consultation with her, Amy said she was getting out of surgery.

And she told Patsy the story. Amy did not turn up for work two days in a row. Concerned colleagues went to her apartment. She was sleeping off the effects of too much alcohol. And she resigned on the spot. The good news is that Amy became a different person once she left that hospital department. She found a much more satisfying job in medicine and is now happier and more fulfilled in her career. Unfortunately, the culture and bullying in this department meant the loss of a good female surgeon to the profession.

## What you can do right now to make a change

### EXAMINE YOUR STRESSORS AND COPING STRATEGIES

Identify what fills your bucket. Write down all these things that cause you stress in your daily world of work. Then identify your taps. Think about what strategies you use to reduce the impact of these stressors. Do you use problem-focused strategies or emotionally focused strategies? How helpful are they for you? Is there something else you could consider?

The benefits that can follow are that you know yourself better and can make changes. Are there any false taps? Are there coping strategies that you use that might alleviate the stress in the short term but increase it and fill the stress bucket in the long term?

## MIND THE GAP AND RESPOND WITH RESILIENT CHOICES

Increasing self-awareness increases resilience and your ability to respond well to stress. Thousands of years ago, even the Oracle of Delphi advised: *"know thyself"*. From a resilience point of view, this self-awareness encompasses an awareness of your strengths and limitations, your needs and drives, and your emotions. Self-awareness around stress is being aware of your body's responses to stress, which might include feelings, desires, and urges to act. It also includes awareness of your thoughts and feelings and how the mind-body relationship plays out in practice.

Knowing thyself is a foundational pillar of resilience and wellbeing. This self-awareness gives you time to pause and consider before acting. In addition, increasing awareness gives you the opportunity for more choice and control in how you respond.

For example, let's take thoughts. If thoughts are operating outside of your awareness, such as common thinking traps, they can significantly influence your emotions and behaviours. On the other hand, if you can bring them into your window of attention, then there's an opportunity for you to consider these thoughts before choosing, deciding, and acting. In short, increasing your self-awareness gives you choice and control because you increase the gap between stimulus and response.

Viktor Frankl, a Holocaust survivor and author of *Man's Search for Meaning,* said that *"between stimulus and response there is a space. In that space is our power to choose our response. In our response lies our growth and our freedom."* This quote reminds me of what a friend once said – when our feet slip, we can regain our balance. But unfortunately, when our tongue slips, it isn't easy to undo what's been said.

There are two ways – formal and informal – to grow the space between stimulus and response. Formal practices to foster awareness are through mindfulness-based practices, especially mindfulness-based stress reduction, to cultivate an understanding of your reactions to stress. You might be thinking, *"You are kidding me. You want me to spend hours doing mindfulness?"* We are not suggesting that you spend hours on this, and we'll show you some quick and easy practices shortly.

There are also informal practices to build resilience on the run. We'll show you activities you can do to promote this. For example, we like using a focused diaphragmatic breath at key moments throughout the day and when asking reflective questions.

When stressed, you are likely to experience early warning signs such as irritability, fatigue, or mood swings. Many doctors we work with push through these physical, emotional, or cognitive warning signs and hope that their natural adaptive response will bring them back to baseline. However, over time this is likely to increase stress and make it more challenging to address the stressor and your response to it. There's also a missed learning opportunity to identify the stressor and develop a way to respond healthily.

Viktor Frankl states, *"Everything can be taken from a man but one thing: the last of the human freedoms – to choose one's attitude in any given set of circumstances, to choose one's own way."*

Think of the wisest people that you've known. Once you have a picture of that person in your mind's eye, consider some of the qualities that make them wise. For example, these qualities might be that they have educated themselves, are disciplined, patient, take instructions humbly, or know how to control themselves when others are losing their heads. One quality of wise people is that they are likely to use the space between stimulus and response in an effective manner.

## What you can do right now to make a change

BREAK YOUR HABITUAL RESPONSE TO A STRESSOR BY ASKING THIS QUESTION

Next time you feel your blood temperature rise, take a deep breath and ask how a wise person would respond.

The benefit that follows is that by merely asking this question, you increase the space between stimulus and response. And reflecting on what a wise person would do paints a picture of an answer that might break your habitual response to this stressor.

# DO COMMON THINKING TRAPS HIJACK YOU?

You probably know someone who makes mountains out of molehills or who always imagines the worst consequences, although they are not remotely possible. These people are caught in thinking traps.

Here's an example of how mental processes affect emotions and behaviour. Imagine three young doctors waiting on the corner for cabs to go to work at their various hospitals or clinics. An empty cab comes along. The cab driver looks at them, waves, and keeps driving without stopping.

The first doctor thinks, *"Oh, no, I'm going to be late to work again. If my supervisor finds out, they might give me a bad report. If I get another bad report, then I'm not going to pass this term."* This thinking is an example of catastrophic thinking that will generate unnecessary stress and anxiety.

The second doctor thinks, *"I got to the corner to hail my cab 15 minutes ago but no matter what I do, I can't seem to start my shift on time. I'm so hopeless."* This doctor's thoughts revolve around a lack of agency – no matter what they do, their actions don't affect the outcome. This is an example of an overgeneralisation and is likely to lead to a degree of helplessness, sadness, or even depression.

The third doctor thinks that the cab driver does not like them, even when there's little evidence of this effect. This is an example of mind-reading, which can lead to a loss of self-esteem and sadness.

As you can see, the event had the same input from the environment, but there were three very different outputs. These are known as consequences and can be behaviours or emotions. The first doctor felt anxiety, the second a level of helplessness, and the third a degree of sadness. These emotions also influence their behaviour.

How we interpret inputs from the environment matters, so modifying cognitions involves recognising your thoughts and asking yourself if you are falling into any common thinking traps.

People often think that external events determine the feelings and emotions they experience. For example, we often hear, *"The exam made me so anxious,"* or *"My partner made me so angry."* However, our thoughts are the links between these external events and how they made us feel. For example, if you have the thought that something bad might happen, then you'll likely feel anxiety, or if you think that somebody has violated your rights, then you'll likely feel angry.

Our thoughts influence our emotions and behaviour. It is easy to fall into negative thinking patterns and spend time bullying ourselves, dwelling on the past, or worrying about the future. Now, of course, 95% of the time, you might deal with the stressors that life throws at you, but there might be clutch moments for you where your thinking lets you down.

Falling into common thinking traps increases your chances of stress, depression, or burnout.

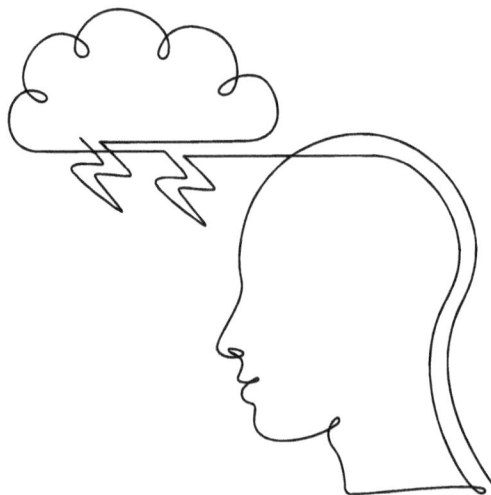

Some thinking traps that we've found particularly common for junior doctors, especially in their lead-up to exams, are black and white thinking, catastrophising, emotional reasoning, mind-reading, and overgeneralisation. Below are explanations of these common thinking traps and some examples that doctors often say to themselves.

| THINKING TRAP | DEFINITION | EXAMPLES |
|---|---|---|
| Black and white thinking | When you view a situation in only two categories instead of a continuum. | "I'm going to fail again" or "I just can't concentrate" or "I haven't got time." |
| Catastrophising | You predict the future negatively without considering other, more likely possibilities. | "What if I fail" or "If I fail, I will never become a good doctor." |
| Emotional reasoning | You think something must be true because you "feel" it so strongly – ignoring or discounting other evidence to the contrary. | "Nobody is helping me" or "I know I do a lot of things OK, but I still feel like a failure." |
| Mind-reading | You believe you know what others are thinking and don't consider other, more likely possibilities. | "My consultant doesn't like me because he failed my last term." |
| Overgeneralisation | You make sweeping negative conclusions that go far beyond the current situation. | "There's too much to learn" or (because you feel uncomfortable with the volume of work) "I don't have what it takes to become a doctor." |

As the Greek Stoic philosopher, Epictetus mentions, *"People are not disturbed by events themselves, but rather by the views they take of them."* Falling into thinking traps affects wellbeing, stress, anxiety, and depression. Once you know thinking traps are common for you, it's harder to fall for them. Instead, you recognise them and avoid them more often.

For example, we knew a doctor who was quite optimistic about life but became the oracle of doom around exam time. And this was her third attempt. Knowing that she was falling into the thinking trap of catastrophic thinking allowed her to develop strategies to challenge this, increase her wellbeing and reduce her stress. She passed!

# What you can do right now to make a change

LEARN HOW TO GET OUT OF A THINKING TRAP

In our experience, doctors try to get out of the thinking trap by telling themselves to stop thinking that way. But this is not a good approach to take. For example, if we ask you not to think of a pink elephant, you are likely to think of a pink elephant. Pushing thoughts away is like pulling a rubber band, they tend to pop back into your mind with a snap. It is much better to consider the evidence and challenge the thinking trap.

1. IDENTIFY YOUR THOUGHTS. Consider some of your stressful events and see if you can identify the thoughts running through your mind. What are your emotions? What are your behaviours? How do you cope?

2. IDENTIFY THE THINKING TRAP. Considering your thoughts, do you notice whether you are falling into a particular thinking trap? Review the list above of some common thinking traps that junior doctors can fall into.

3. CHALLENGE THE THINKING TRAP. For example, you might want to examine the evidence. If you made a mistake at the hospital, you might automatically think, *"I can't do anything right; I must be a terrible doctor!"* When this thought comes up, can you challenge it by asking, "What is the evidence that both supports and does not support this thought"? When you consider these questions, you might notice that you received a compliment from your supervisor for a job well done at work last week.

4. PUT THE THINKING TRAP INTO PERSPECTIVE. Has this happened in the past? What was the outcome? What's the worst-case scenario and how could you deal with it? How important will this be in a week, a month, or a year? If this were to happen to a friend, what would you say?

Once you have worked through your thinking trap, try to find a balanced thought to replace those old thinking traps.

The benefit that follows is that you have a way to consider and make a change.

## MINDFULNESS IS HAVING ITS MOMENT

Mindfulness is having its moment with a wealth of new research that has explored an ancient practice. Numerous studies on mindfulness have shown that mindfulness reduces rumination and stress; increases working memory, focus, cognitive flexibility, and enhances relationships. In a meta-analysis that explored 39 studies, published in the *Journal of Consulting and Clinical Psychology* (2010), Hoffman and colleagues found that mindfulness reduced anxiety and improved mood symptoms. The evidence-based literature shows that mindfulness alleviates symptoms of poor mental health and aids psychological wellbeing.

Mindfulness is not about dressing up in monk robes and living the life of a hermit. Instead, according to Jon Kabat-Zinn in his book *Mindfulness for Beginners: Reclaiming the Present Moment – and Your Life*, it is an *"awareness, cultivated by paying attention in a sustained and particular way: on purpose, in the present moment, and non-judgementally."* This definition of mindfulness has three critical parts: the intention, attention, and attitude you bring to the practice.

Mindfulness-based programs reduce stress and burnout of otherwise healthy individuals. For example, they have been used in the workplace to reduce symptoms of burnout for nurses and physicians and reduce the stress of medical students. However, the busy schedules of junior doctors can often mean that the length of time to practice mindfulness meditation can be limited.

According to a meta-analysis that looked at multiple studies on brief mindfulness practices for healthcare providers, mindfulness for as little as five to 10 minutes a day can impact healthcare providers' stress and reduce burnout.

## What you can do right now to make a change

EXPLORE THESE MINDFULNESS TECHNIQUES

Close your eyes and bring your attention to your breath. Notice the rise and fall of your chest and abdomen. Also, notice the breath moving in and out of the nostrils.

Now imagine a slow-moving stream or river. You're sitting on the bank of this river. And you are watching the boats sailing past. Each of these boats has a different size, shape, and colour. Each represents a thought, a wish, a feeling, or a bodily sensation. You're watching these thoughts, feelings, and sensations coming down the river. Try not to jump into the boat or push the boat away. Instead, simply observe the boat and then let it move on until it disappears. Let all come and go.

Did you notice any thoughts, feelings, or bodily sensations riding in the boats? Were you able to let the boats float by? Did you get into any of the boats or rafts? If so, which ones and why? Looking at your thoughts and feelings differently, you can choose whether to get "caught up" in these or let go of your attachment to them.

There are two meditations that we recommend to clients. Both can be beneficial with as little as five minutes' practice.

The first is mindfulness meditation. This originates from Buddhist teachings and is the most popular type of meditation in the west. In mindfulness meditation, you let your thoughts pass through your mind. You observe them without judgement, like leaves floating down a stream.

The second is focused meditation, which involves bringing your attention or focus to one of your five senses – the most common is breathing. When your mind wanders to the thoughts that you have, you bring it gently back to the focus of the breath.

The benefit of these short meditations is that they can fit into your schedule and create habits for increased opportunities to practise mindfulness.

## SOCIAL FACTORS THAT INCREASE RESILIENCE

Keeping the other areas of your life going increases resilience. Kell first heard of the Four Burner Theory as an analogy of life in an article by David Sedaris popularised by James Clear, author of *Atomic Habits*. In the Four Burner Theory, each burner represents a significant quadrant of your life. For example, one burner represents your health, one burner represents your work, one represents your family, and one represents your friends. In the Four Burner Theory, to be successful with one of your burners, you need to turn off one of your other burners. To be highly successful, you need to turn off two of your burners.

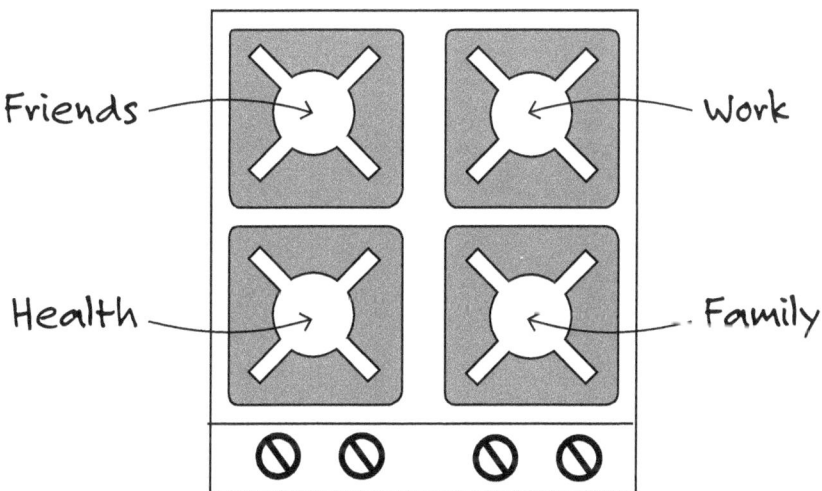

According to this theory, to be a successful doctor, you need to consider turning off one or two of your burners that relate to family, friends, or health. Our initial thought when first coming across the Four Burner Theory was, *"Can I bypass this? What burner do I need to turn off?"* Although the Four Burner Theory provides an apt summary of the constraints to how much time we can invest into each of those areas, we don't wholeheartedly agree with the idea that the time spent in one area of life is a trade-off to other areas, especially when it comes to the resilience and performance of doctors. What would you turn off so that you can focus on your work and study as a doctor? Would it be family? Would it be your health? Would it be friends?

## We argue that balance can make all four burners grow brighter for a junior doctor.

Let's work through an example. Let's say that you decide to turn off the burner of health to increase the flame of work. By turning off the burner of health, you consciously choose not to focus your time and effort on health and wellbeing. Yet, good sleep, good exercise, and good nutrition are core pillars of resilience. As we've mentioned in earlier chapters, optimal brain function is supported by a hard-working body, so in this case, the burner of health adds to the flames of work.

In another example, let's consider that you want to manage your stress and health better. You could turn off the flame of friends, but there's an abundant amount of research that highlights that family and friends buffer us from the effects of stress. If we can maintain our relationships with others, we are less prone to stress, anxiety, depression, or burnout. The Four Burner Theory provides a helpful metaphor for the constraints we face and how to get more time in each area of our lives. So what's the best way to handle some of these problems?

# What you can do right now to make a change

CONSIDER THESE OPTIONS FOR KEEPING ALL FOUR
BURNERS GOING

How can you keep all four burners going? Each of those burners contributes to overall performance and overall wellbeing and resilience. Here are a few options:

**Can you outsource any of the burners?** Draw up a list of activities you've done across the last fortnight. Are there activities that you can outsource others to do? For example, if you're a busy doctor, can you outsource parts of your life such as mowing the lawn or cleaning your house to focus on the other burners?

**Consider embracing the constraints.** The Four Burner Theory says that we've got 24 hours a day and that there's a trade-off across each of the burners. Recognising this, how can you maximise the time? If I'm going to work from 9 am to 5 pm, how can I bring the most value to that time? I'm planning to study for two hours a day. How can I get the most from that time? If I'm spending a few hours a day with my loved ones, how can I make that quality time? Consider protecting in advance the important things you do that bring value to other burners, such as exercise or family time.

**The seasons of life.** When Kell was raising three little boys, the burners of friends and health were turned off because he was focused on feeding and raising a young family. The focus of the burner might change with the period of life that you're in. Each junior doctor is in a season of life, and it's important to recognise this. While you might not be able to turn down the burner on your family, especially if you've got three little children, do you have support around you to maintain the different burners? Perhaps you're going through a particularly tense time at work. Do you need to organise support and let others know?

CONSIDER SHARING THE FLAME ACROSS THE DIFFERENT BURNERS. Can colleagues become friends? Can you work out with your friends? Can you combine any of your burners so that spending time on one burner does not take away from time on another burner?

The benefits are as follows: When it comes to resilience and performance, one flame can build the other flame to complement and grow each other. For example, promoting health improves work and study performance. Resilience and good performance are supported by having balance across each of those different areas of your life.

## SUMMARY

Jettison your old thinking about resilience – the strategy of toughening up and pushing through is not a sustainable way to manage your stress and overwhelming thoughts. There are many more effective strategies to increase your resilience and wellbeing. These include:

- identifying your causes of stress and increasing your awareness of how you respond to this stress
- recognising the common thinking traps that you might fall into and how to challenge this
- adding some mindfulness-based techniques into your day
- finding ways to keep your four burners alight.

If we're going to dedicate more time for resilience and spend time ensuring that our four burners stay alight, then we need to think about saving time somewhere else. In the next chapter, we will look at how to study smarter, not longer. We will look at how to study shorter and get more retention from the content you're taking in.

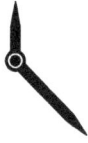

# CHAPTER FOUR

# STUDY SMARTER, NOT LONGER

In this chapter, we first challenge various ideas about how to study. There is a familiar concept known as the forgetting curve within memory research. We will look at flattening the forgetting curve to remember more of what you study. Then we will look at ways you can study smarter, not longer. We get that this is challenging or terrifying for you. You might have failed in the past, and your whole being might be screaming, *"I have to study more. Show us how to find more hours."* But here we are, saying, *"Study less."* By studying smarter, you can spend less time at your desk and retain more information. Next, we'll look at how to get more out of your content as you read. Then we will look at acing your learning by studying less and testing more. Finally, we will examine the spacing effect to ramp up retention to make the study content stick.

Most people don't know how to study. We know that this is a bold statement to make, given that this is a book written for junior doctors who have largely aced every exam they have taken.

For junior doctors, there are large swathes of reading each day to get through your exams. The volume is quite different from high school and medical school, where exams are nearly always on the semester just finished. When we ask the doctors we work with how they study at home, many tell us that they re-read their books and make copious notes. But when we ask, *"Is this the best way to retain and apply the information?"* they often tell us they don't know.

The answer is no. While re-reading increases the total amount of information encoded and helps with processing the ideas to increase the memory of a topic, it doesn't help you apply and evaluate the content that's so necessary for your exams and your profession as a doctor.

Some doctors point out that they adopt the highlighting strategy for essential points of information. Highlighting has some crucial functions. It helps a written word pop out, which can be helpful when you want to come back to the essential points. However, it is likely to fall over for junior doctors due to the large quantity of material you need to cover. Each chapter and paragraph is packed with information, and the consequence is that you may find that you have highlighted large sections of content. When we ask, *"Is this a good way to learn important concepts?"* again, they say they don't know.

This is what we mean by "most people have not been shown how to study".

You wouldn't use old technology on patients, so don't use outdated study methods on yourself. The consequence of using outdated study methods is that you are likely to be studying for longer hours than neccessary.

There's much opportunity to use the brain in an optimal way to synthesise and integrate the material into their long-term memory and reduce feelings of being overwhelmed.

# FLATTENING THE FORGETTING CURVE – STRATEGIES TO MAKE YOUR LEARNING STICK

You're probably more familiar with forgetting than you think. Was it Alexander the Great who won the battle of Issus in Southern Anatolia? What was Macbeth angry about in Shakespeare's play? What are the first few numbers in the pi formulation, how do we use that to calculate the circumference of a circle? All these things we learned in high school, but their answers now elude us, even after studying half our lives in these areas. This is a universal experience because we all forget, and you can plot the rate you forget with the forgetting curve.

Many doctors who visit us tend to study for long hours to absorb the material then get frustrated when they can't recall that important fact or process. They know they read it not long ago, and they are hyper-aware that forgetting is a costly mistake because it could be in the exam, and everything's riding on this. We often tell them that when you understand why you forget, you can thwart the forgetting and make sure that what you learn sticks.

The earliest research done on this was by German psychologist Hermann Ebbinghaus way back in the 1880s, who produced the forgetting curve. His research is still widely used and highly regarded. A research team in 2015 reproduced his findings and found that his methods and theories still hold.

The forgetting curve refers to the rate of loss of new information over time. The graph below shows the rate of forgetting and that memories weaken over time. If we learn something new and then don't take any time to relearn that information, we remember less.

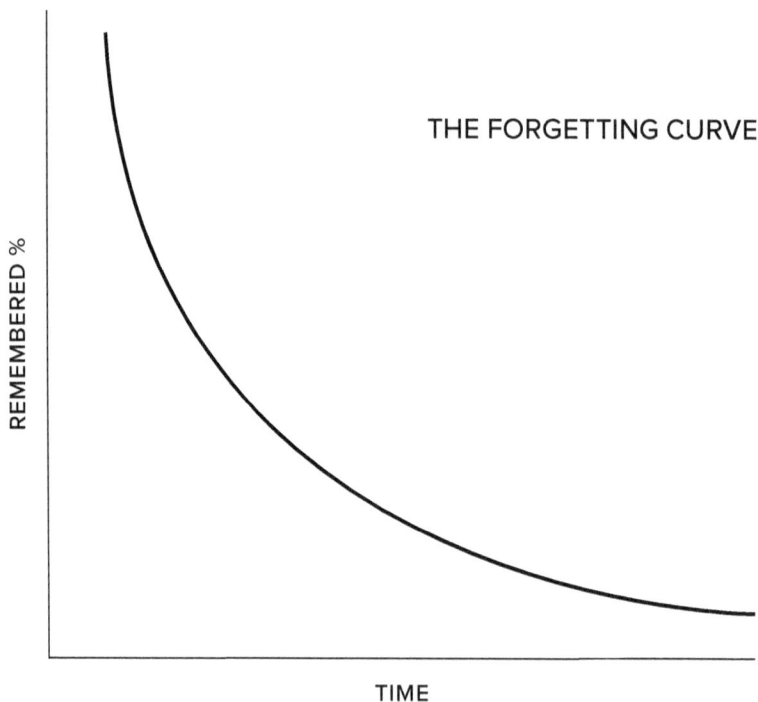

THE FORGETTING CURVE

REMEMBERED %

TIME

Ebbinghaus's forgetting curve has implications for your study strategy. More than half of memory loss occurs within the first hour. Most of the material that will be forgotten is done within the first eight hours, then it steadies out. A day after you're attending a lecture, reading a chapter or article, you'll have lost approximately 75% of what was learned. The forgetting curve is a natural process, but it has significant implications for strategies associated with your study.

## WHAT'S THE EVIDENCE?

In a study of 129 students by Ebersbach and Nazari, published in 2020 in the *Journal of Applied Research in Memory and Cognition*, students were put into two groups.

- Group one students were asked to space out their studies on three different days.
- Group two were asked to cram all their study into one day.

The students attended several lectures on specific content for their degree, so they had acquired the relevant skills from a body of lectures. The students needed to practice these skills at home.

Students were tested five weeks later. Students in group one had better memory performance than students in group two. This improved performance was not only for previously practised skills but also for new tasks.

This highlights that spaced practice is a powerful tool for fostering long-term retention and transfer for adults in an authentic educational context.

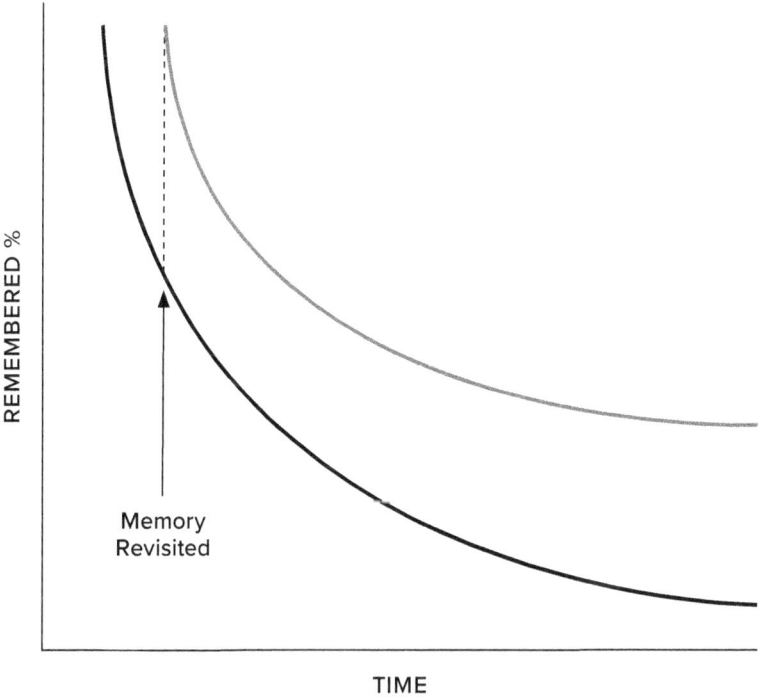

To flatten the forgetting curve, Patsy has learned to change how she gives homework in her first consultation. She used to cram as much information as possible into the hour-long session. This was so that doctors would assimilate the material as soon as possible into their new study plans.

However, at the second consultation, Patsy often found that the instructions were not followed as closely as she would have liked. Doctors had forgotten some of the instructions. She often found to her amusement that doctors had been quite creative in the way they interpreted the homework based on what they remembered. Patsy now slows down, gives fewer instructions at each consultation, and makes sure the client takes notes. She now finds that the tasks she has set are being more accurately remembered and performed.

## SPACED LEARNING

Spaced learning, also known as distributed practice, involves reviewing information over several periods rather than all at once. Kell likes to think of spaced learning like building the brick wall at the front of his house. If he lays the bricks in a rush and doesn't let the mortar between each brick dry, his front wall will not be very good quality. What spaced learning does is allow the mental mortar time to dry.

While there are many mechanisms by which spacing benefits long-term retention, a key one is that spacing allows your brain to consolidate information, so it's easier to retrieve when necessary.

Imagine one junior doctor sitting down for seven hours to learn concepts in their books. Another junior doctor spends one hour each day for a week. Which doctor is most likely to walk away with greater retention? The research says that the second doctor's regular study and retrieval of information may have strengthened the neural pathways, undergirded memory, and allowed more opportunities to practise what has been learned – either consciously or unconsciously.

Each time you revisit the content, the benefit is that you are flattening the forgetting curve until it effectively becomes a straight line like below.

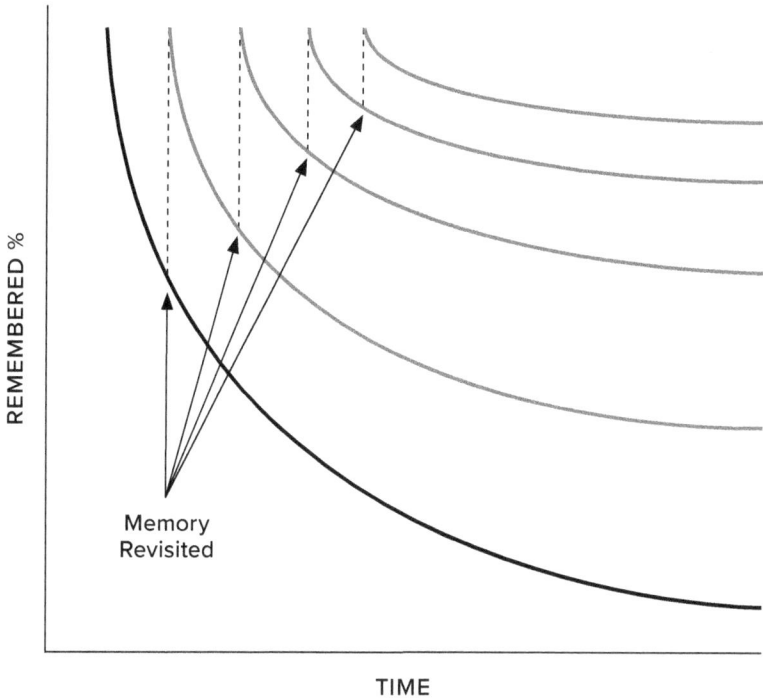

## What you can do right now to make a change

CREATE A SPACED STUDY SCHEDULE

Now that you know you lose 75% of your memories in 24 hours, here's how to disrupt it. Schedule learning time like this:

- Allocate time (an hour) to study a topic.

- 24 hours later, block out 15 minutes to review it.

- Seven days later, block out 15 minutes for a review.

- 30 days later, block out 15 minutes for a review.

Now you've flattened the forgetting curve.

## TO ACE YOUR LEARNING, STUDY LESS AND TEST MORE

The next thing you can add to your study smarter strategy is regular testing. Testing is known as retrieval practice within the literature. A meta-analysis of several hundred studies published by John Dunlosky and colleagues in the 2013 issue of the *Psychological Science in the Public Interest* has shown that practice testing helps students retrieve information and produces more significant gains in learning than simply studying.

One reason why testing improves recall is that you're extracting the information out of your memory.

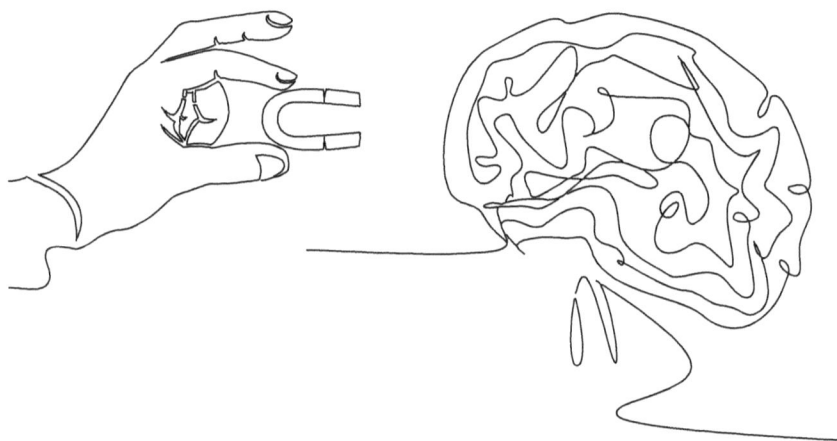

It seems counterintuitive that this retrieval of memory aids you in understanding the content; however, testing asks your brain to remember cue information. As you reach back into your memory banks, you also organise the information or reconstruct the knowledge and identify strategies for retrieving that information out of your long-term memory. So you are better able to recall this information in the future. In short, you are practising what you need to do later in your exam.

This approach increases your recall and thwarts the forgetting curve. How cool is that? That's more time with the kids, your friends, and your loved ones.

## WHAT'S THE EVIDENCE?

In one study, published by Jeffrey Karpicke and Janell Blunt in the 2011 issue of the *American Association for the Advancement of Science,* science students were put into one of the following groups.

- Group one studied the science text just once.
- Group two was repeatedly studying over four time periods.
- Group three studied the content and then created an elaborative concept map of the content.
- Group four studied the text in an initial study period and then did a practice test.

The total amount of time was matched across the conditions. It was found that group four, those who read a science passage then took a test asking them to recall what they had read, retained 50% more information a week later than students who used the other methods.

# What you can do right now to make a change

## TRY THIS TESTING METHOD IN YOUR NEXT STUDY SESSION

As you read your content, write several questions related to that topic and number them. Don't answer them now; put them away for a few days.

As part of your next session on this topic, put some time aside for your testing. Go over the questions you wrote down and see if you can answer them verbally. The type of testing and the length of testing will vary, and this largely depends on how far away from the exams you are. The point of this exercise is simply to increase long-term

**retention via moving from a passive process of reading to an active process of testing.**

Two things to note here, which we'll talk about in later chapters:

1.  If you test at night when you're tired, it's as though you're practising exam components under pressure. You can then allocate study sessions the next day to go over some of the errors in your testing.
2.  Spacing practice is like a burger, and retrieval practice is like chips. Both taste delicious, but when you combine them, the real magic happens. It's the same with memory. Combining spacing and retrieval practice is a perfect strategy for increasing retention.

## HOW TO GET MORE OUT OF THE CONTENT YOU READ

Have you ever read a page of your medical text only to get to the end of the page and realise that you have no idea what you have just read? One reason for this is that reading is a passive process. Successful readers who retain information use active reading strategies for deeper engagement and involvement.

If we asked you to remember N-X-Y-Z-A or P-E-A-R-S, you're far more likely to recall pears when asked later. You're less likely to remember nonsense syllables with little or no meaning, which conforms to the forgetting curve. Reading is essential to knowledge acquisition. It's a must-do activity to learn the information you need to pass your exams. However, reading comes in two broad flavours – passive and active.

Passive reading is when the person reads the content but does not engage with it or absorbs very little of it. In the passive reading process, they would be unlikely to stop and think about whether they understand the content or take the time to reflect and evaluate what they have read.

Active reading involves a deeper level of engagement with the text, both before and during reading. The active reader will often stop to monitor their understanding of the text and take time to reflect upon and evaluate what they have read. This style of reading increases comprehension and memory retention.

From what we know about junior doctors, even if they do remember and understand the content they've read from their medical text, this does not mean that they know how to apply, analyse, or evaluate the material – the very expertise required of a doctor. Unlike active reading, passive reading provides familiarity and could give you the illusion that you know the content.

If you adopt the active reading strategy,
then you'll study more effectively and hold
more information in your mind.

## PEDRO'S STORY, TOLD BY PATSY

*Pedro, a basic physician trainee, thought he knew the content because he did hours of passive study reading his notes. He was angry that he failed his written exams on the first go (all multiple-choice questions). What more could he do?*

*I introduced him to a form of active reading. In each of his 50-minute study sessions, Pedro was to select five or six facts, the sort that might come up on multiple-choice questions. Next, he was to write these facts down word for word on a sheet of paper. Then, he was to flip the sheet over and write as a heading the topic he was studying in that 50-minute session. Finally, he was to write a question for each of the facts that would regurgitate the fact, then put the sheet of paper away.*

I advised him not to try to answer the questions for 24 to 36 hours, as it was likely the facts would still be in working memory. About four or five days later, after a day (or night) shift, Pedro was to retrieve his piece of paper and record the answers to these questions into an audio app on his phone (and of course, not look at the answers on the other side!) Then he was to mark his answers immediately. First, he was to turn over the question sheet, listen to his answer on the phone, then give it a score from one to 10 for the accuracy of the content. He was to do this with all questions.

Then he was to play back the answers again and listen to the voice tone. Was it confident? Was it clear? Did he mumble? Was he tentative? And he was to give a score from 1 to 10 as to how his voice sounded.

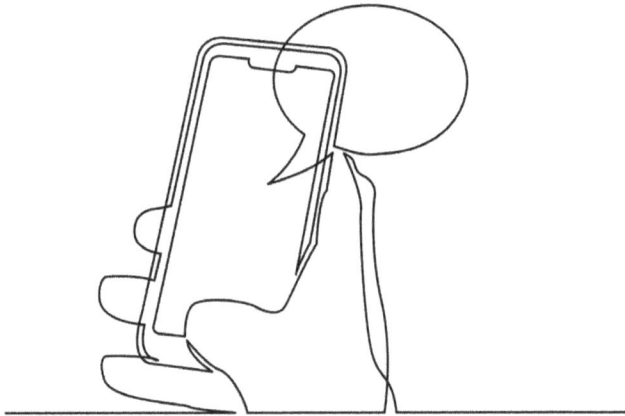

I suggested that Pedro pretend it's a colleague he's listening to. After all, nobody likes the sound of their voice. Any low scores, whether for content or voice tone, were noted as they indicated he did not know the material well enough for an exam.

I advised him not to read around the answers with low scores immediately after marking them. Instead, he should allocate future study sessions to reading and understanding the material when he was fresh.

He was to do this active reading for each of his 50-minute study *sessions. So, if, for example, he had seven study sessions in a week, then he would need to mark a sheet of five or six questions each night of the week. It would only take 15 minutes or so to record and mark each sheet.*

*Pedro was quite enthusiastic about active reading, particularly when he realised the benefits: there was revision of previous reading, multiple-choice questions in his exams were made up of facts just like these, and he realised it was good practice for viva exams as he became used to the sound of his voice. Pedro passed his written exams at the next sitting.*

## What you can do right now to make a change

MOVE FROM PASSIVE TO ACTIVE READING

There are several steps you can take to move from passive to active reading.

1. **Know your purpose.** It's helpful to be clear on the chapter objectives before you read. What are you reading the chapter in the medical text for? Are you clear on the learning outcomes of the chapter? Most books have these written at the front of the chapter. If you read these and then read the chapter, you are more likely to read with purpose and retain the content.

2. **Skim the chapter you plan to read.** A proper skim of the chapter primes the memory as you read over some subsections or subsection titles and helps you remember what you're going to read.

3. **Ask and answer questions.** As you're reading, take a moment to ask yourself questions such as: What are the text's key ideas? What's new to us here? How could we define this concept? How do these ideas relate to what we already know? Consider turning the chapter headings and subheadings into questions and answering them as you read. Form questions as you read, and then put them aside and answer them later. See the above section on spacing and how this flattens the forgetting curve.

Use this quizzing to identify strengths and weaknesses and focus your study on this. The harder it is for you to recall ideas or answers from memory, the greater the benefit. Effortful retrieval makes for more robust learning and retention. If you make an error, that's okay if you correct your answer. Many readers will highlight texts, but retrieval is better if you can build questions around the content of the text. As a Chinese scholar, Wang Yongzhi once wrote, *"If you read or do research with small questions in mind, you learn small things. If you do so with big questions in mind, you learn big things. If you do so with no questions in mind, you learn nothing."*

**4. Ask yourself if you can connect this information to what you already know**. For example, when learning about social norms in psychology, you are much more able to remember your learning if you connect this concept to something practical in our lives, such as waiting in a queue.

If you take these four steps, you move from a passive to an active reader, with the benefits that accrue with each step.

## SUMMARY

You now have the information to change your study habits to study smarter, not longer. Your study needs to be shorter in length, more focused, and involve testing of material. Consider your syllabus and the other things going on in your life. Plan out a new way of studying that involves spacing out your practice and dedicated spots to test your knowledge. When reading your text, read with purpose and look for questions that you can test yourself on later.

We've talked largely about ways to enhance your study, but the rubber hits the road when we apply more of these ideas to your specific exam components.

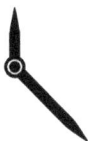

# CHAPTER FIVE

# TRAIN FOR KNOWLEDGE ACQUISITION

Doctors often fail the knowledge components of written exams by small margins. This chapter will look at the different types of questions and how to close that margin. It is possible that some doctors are not using the testing techniques that are appropriate for different types of questions. We'll look at questions based on recognition memory. We will cover learning to differentiate the study and testing of objective questions from comprehension questions and talk about resources. Colleges don't release objective questions, so we will give you some suggestions on where you can get these resources. Testing your knowledge and lots of test repetition is the key to success. We will be applying deliberate practice techniques that you learned in Chapter Four to master answering objective questions. Lastly, we will discuss how priming the brain for subsequent learning comes from struggling to retrieve information.

In her 1979 article, "Recognition Memory for Chess Positions" in the *American Journal of Psychology*, Sarah Goldin defines recognition memory as the ability to identify a familiar stimulus or a situation encountered previously. Recognition memory is most important when answering the parts of exams with objective or knowledge-type questions. These objective questions are based on your ability to recognise facts as they are written in your textbooks or notes. Multiple-choice questions are the most popular type of objective questions. You have plausible choices which happen to be incorrect.

Recognition is a cognitive ability that makes it possible to recover stored information and compare it to the presented information. The presentation of a familiar outside stimulus provides a cue that the information has been seen before. For example, recognising a fact you had previously read in the recommended text provides a cue for you. According to Henry Roediger and Jeffrey Karpicke, in their 2006 article on test-enhanced learning in *Psychological Science*, how easily information can be retrieved from memory depends on three factors:

- How often have you encountered that information?

- How recently have you tested it?

- How much is it related to the current context?

You need to regularly practise test questions using these factors to prove to yourself that you can rely on it and then trust it. In other words, have you encountered the information on many occasions, perhaps in texts, presentations, research articles, notes? Have you or somebody else had to answer a question on this topic in tutorials, clinical rounds, or study groups? Is this information you recognise and relate to when doing handovers or when treating patients?

*Testing and retesting subject matter increases your ability to recognise information and facts.*

## FACTS – USE THAT RECOGNITION MEMORY

Facts are the answers to objective questions. You must train your recognition memory to get them right. You need to learn and recognise basic facts on each topic if you have objective questions in your exams. Facts in the textbooks are often used word for word in the multiple-choice answers to objective questions. Your recognition memory uses the words in the textbook as a prompt or cue to remind you which is the correct answer. It helps if you read the required textbooks, when available, so you recognise the answer when you see it.

The risk is that you could be tempted to rote learn rather than read around answers for understanding. As discussed in Chapter Four, when you make notes, you improve your comprehension, which also helps with recognition memory. Write questions that will regurgitate facts that you can later test yourself on. This helps recognition because it strengthens your ability to use the cues, which we will discuss in more detail later.

*Remember that testing yourself on the material you have read, even if you don't get the answers right, still helps the brain to learn.*

To master recognition memory, read the textbook, make notes, and test yourself. This is the active process we discussed in the last chapter.

Learning facts and retaining them in your memory requires repetitive testing to train your recognition memory. The more you train, the more you retain. Space the training out to increase retaining and recognise the cues for choosing the correct answers.

Over the years, we've met doctors who try to memorise the answers to common questions. Mahoud, who worked full-time, had a young family, and usually studied at night or whenever he had a break. After testing and marking his answers, he tried to memorise the correct answers. Being time-poor and not having many resources readily available, he seldom searched in the textbooks for explanations of the correct answers. This meant that his ability to select the correct answer from several plausible answers was limited. Unfortunately, this method did not work well for Mahoud. He failed at his next attempt at the exam. He then changed the way he studied and searched for explanations of the correct answers. He was relieved to pass the exam a few months later.

## COLLECTING RESOURCES FOR OBJECTIVE QUESTIONS

Objective questions are not generally shared after exams by colleges as they are challenging to construct. You need to seek out examples of objective questions in your specialty from wherever possible. Study groups and hospital tutorial groups often make up multiple-choice questions from recommended texts based on various topics. They write appropriate responses and explanations and share these.

Some specialties tend to rely on black banks of questions. These are questions remembered by candidates immediately after exams and written down. They are later shared with others. There is a good chance the wording of the questions is not the same. Often study groups will go over black banks and re-word the questions and answers to increase the accuracy.

You could purchase a bank of questions or share the cost of a bank of questions with a study buddy. You could also ask previous trainees who have now completed their exams to see if they have any spare multiple-choice questions from tutorials they used to attend. Or perhaps they may have practice banks of questions that they no longer use. Because this type of study is based on recognition memory it is essential to have a variety of resources and test your knowledge regularly. If you are posted to a regional hospital, it is important to maintain connections with colleagues in the main tertiary hospitals. And don't be afraid to ask them for resources, which are often sadly lacking in the regional hospitals.

## KATY'S STORY, TOLD BY KELL

*Katy was a basic physical trainee (BPT) in a major tertiary hospital whose first two written exams were based on multiple-choice questions (MCQs). At her first attempt at the exam, she failed. After questioning, I realised Katy did not test herself regularly. Instead, she relied on doing plenty of study, mostly at night after work. I changed Katy's study time to weekend mornings, and every night after work asked her to test MCQs under exam conditions. She then borrowed a bank of questions from a previous trainee and was able to sort them into different topics. I asked her to test on topics that she hadn't revised for a while. She was then to mark for accuracy and note the percentage she got right in a diary. Anything wrong, she was to note and read around the topic at her next study session. A few nights later, when the material she studied was out of working memory, Katy retested the same MCQs again.*

*Katy liked the structure of testing, study, and further testing. She found it motivating to see her percentages of correct answers on topics increase. On her second attempt, she passed the written exam.*

# What you can do right now to make a change

## CREATE A STUDY GROUP

Form a weekly online study group with other doctors in your specialty from various hospitals. This can be a helpful, collaborative process in the weeks and months before an exam. The study group members can then create an action plan based on finding the answers and explanations for multiple-choice questions. Each group member is expected to find the answers and explanations for a specific number of multiple-choice questions each week, which they then share. This involves each group member searching through the textbooks and their notes to find the correct answers to each question they were given.

Sharing this information cuts down the time required by each doctor to search for correct answers, and each person develops a bank of answers.

Each week, the study group then pools all their multiple-choice questions and tests themselves under exam conditions. Ideally, they do this before they have even shared the answers. In this way, they test their knowledge before knowing the actual answers.

Then, in their study time at home, they read around the correct answers for all the shared questions they got wrong when they tested themselves in the study group. And a few days later, when the answers are no longer in working memory, they try those same questions again. If you take these actions, the answers are more likely to be correct through recognition memory.

## TRUST YOUR RECOGNITION MEMORY

Junior doctors often tell us that they failed a previous exam attempt because they failed the multiple-choice questions component by half a point or one point. They are disappointed that they failed by such a small margin. We always ask the same question: *"Did you go back and change your answer to any questions?"* The answer is usually yes. However, they often went from a correct answer to a wrong answer by changing that answer. When we asked why they changed the answer, they said they didn't trust their memory when it recognised the familiar fact. So, they tried to analyse it. The more they analysed and thought about it, the more they felt the wrong answer was the correct one. They would then choose another plausible yet ultimately incorrect answer. The other choices look tempting but remember that this is recognition memory. Go with that first choice.

Practise doing 30 multiple-choice questions daily in 30 minutes under exam conditions – in a quiet room with your phone on silent, keeping to the exact time, and with no interruptions or open textbooks on the table.

> Get into the habit of not changing your mind
> after selecting your answer, no matter how
> tempted you are to do so.

And one more thing. It is helpful to cover up the choices while you think about an answer. In this way, you don't get confused by two similar answers. Of course, you can't do this with every question, but it's a valuable tip to use where possible.

Mark your answers and record the percentage you get right in your diary. Record your scores daily. You'll soon see the percentage going up. And those questions that were not correct? Read around the information on that topic in a study session, and a few days later, test yourself on everything you initially got wrong. You might be pleasantly surprised!

## DELIBERATE PRACTICE IS WORTH IT

Study using these methods, which are designed specifically to improve your performance, is called deliberate practice. Deliberate practice pushes you beyond your comfort zone to identify what needs improving and then work on it. Deliberate practice can also be repeated. High repetition leads to consistency. Feedback on results is continuously available, and self-feedback enables you to recognise your strengths and weaknesses.

**ZONES OF LEARNING**

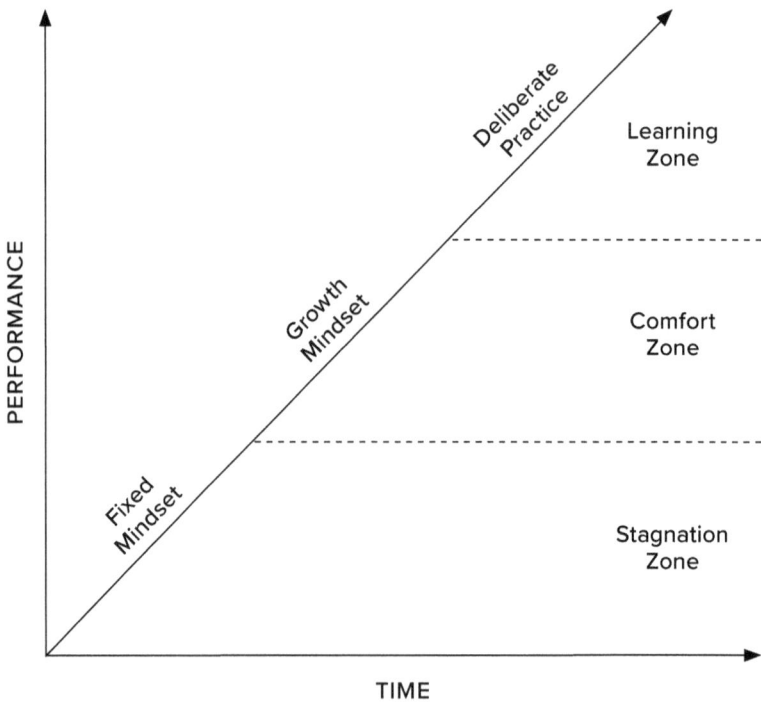

PERFORMANCE

Deliberate Practice

Learning Zone

Growth Mindset

Comfort Zone

Fixed Mindset

Stagnation Zone

TIME

Deliberate practice is highly demanding mentally. It requires effort to focus and concentrate. For example, doing objective questions under exam conditions, assessing, and correcting them, and then repeating the process is mentally tiring but worthwhile. However, it's not much fun. Doing study or testing on the material you know and like is enjoyable. You learn a lot, but you don't always identify problem areas to work on. With deliberate practice you will identify those problem areas. Deliberate practice means working on things you don't like or can't do well, getting feedback, and repeating the process until you improve.

When Patsy was young and learning piano, she wanted to be a reasonably accomplished musician. But, to improve, you don't simply play tunes you like. Patsy always wanted to play songs she liked, and she avoided playing the ones she didn't like. Patsy's grandma kept advising her to spend more time practising the difficult music sheets. But Patsy just wanted to have fun, and when grandma wasn't listening, she practised the piano in her way.

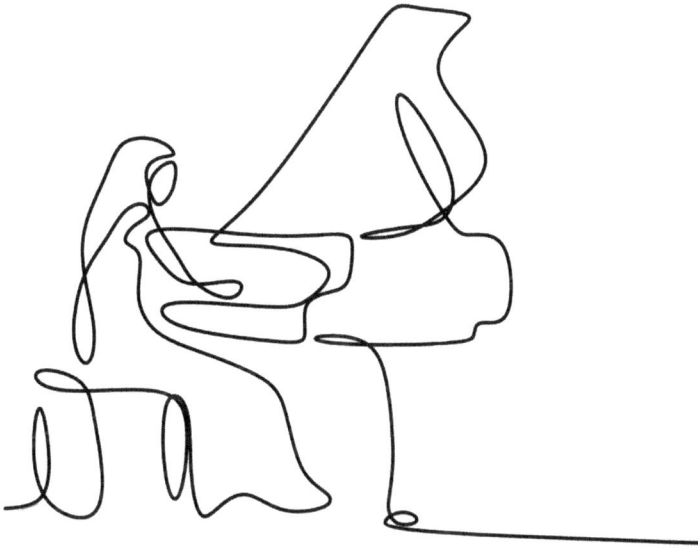

Even though she improved, it didn't allow her to work on problem areas. She learned the hard way, and later wished she'd followed her grandma's wise advice. Young musicians who want to improve will deliberately practise scales, intricate fingering, and fast sections of music. They make a point of doing deliberate practice of those elements regularly. That's what Patsy should have done when she was younger.

# What you can do right now to make a change

## TACKLE THE TOPICS YOU DISLIKE OR AVOID

Tutorial groups often have multiple-choice questions on certain topics. You may have a bank of multiple-choice questions that can be arranged and rearranged to select specific topics. Pick a topic you dislike and tend to avoid. Make a point of practising questions on that topic after work under exam conditions daily until you become proficient with the answers. Attempt to answer the questions in consecutive order. Ignore the answer choices at first by covering them with your hand. We know we've mentioned that previously, but it bears repetition. Read the question carefully and determine the correct answer before reading the answer choices. Then read the answer choices carefully and select the most appropriate answer. You will find there is less confusion if you cover those choices.

# SEARCHING FOR ANSWERS LEADS TO BETTER LEARNING

Struggling to retrieve information primes the brain for subsequent learning, even if you do not always have the correct answers. Sometimes multiple-choice questions banks have the answers but not the explanations. Searching for the answers will help with retention. But be mindful of when you do this. If you practise answering multiple-choice questions after work, only mark them in this testing session but wait until your next study session to read around the material to understand the answers.

It's better to look at the topics and understand the answers when you've had a good sleep, are feeling energetic, and the brain is fresh. You're then more likely to remember the material.

Pretesting before studying the topic prompts the brain to form an early outline that will be filled in with details as learning progresses.

## WHAT'S THE EVIDENCE?

Psychologists Arnold Glass and Mengxue Kang co-authored a research article in 2020, *"Fewer Students are Benefiting from Doing Their Homework: An Eleven-year Study."* Glass and Kang advise to *"always generate the answers for yourself. It will help you do better in the exam".* The article has indicated that searching for answers is a better way to retrieve information from the brain when you later study the topic. This helps to make your learning stick.

Glass and Kang discovered this from analysing homework and the grades on tests given to college students from 2008 to 2017. Glass gave his students a quiz-style online series of homework assignments in which the students answered homework questions about the upcoming material the day before a lecture. They answered similar questions in class and a week later in the exam. Mengxue Kang says, *"if you test yourself, again and again, you will have better performance in the end."* During the most recent two years of the study, when students were asked how they did their homework, students who benefited from homework reported generating their own answers and students who reported copying the answers from another source did not benefit from homework. These findings would suggest that self-testing using multiple-choice questions before studying the topic primes the mind for learning and retention.

It takes a little more time to test, study, and then retest, compared to studying and then testing. You will have better overall results if you test first and struggle to think of the answers.

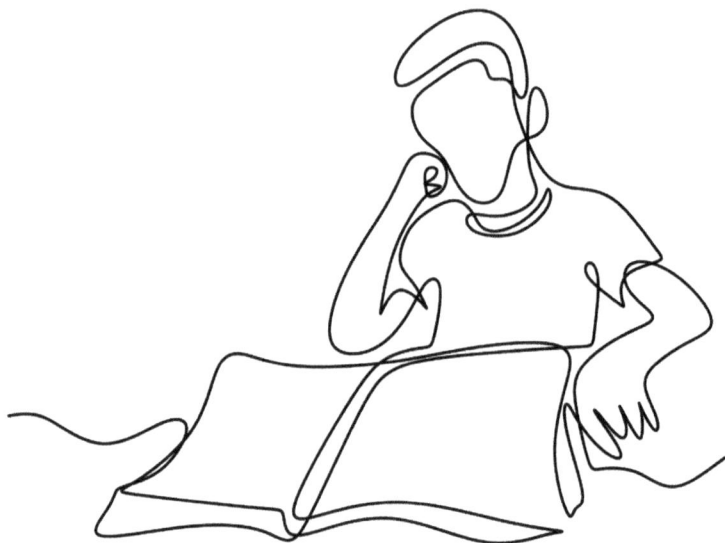

## What you can do right now to make a change

TRY THE TEST-STUDY-RETEST METHOD

So, before you even study a particular topic, test yourself on 30 multiple-choice questions in 30 minutes and record the percentage of correct answers. Don't be disheartened if your score is low. And be pleasantly surprised if you score well! Then study that topic in one of your morning study sessions. Retest again on the same questions, preferably a few days later when the material is no longer in working memory. Again, record the percentage of correct answers.

Compare this test-study-retest with studying first and then testing yourself some days later on 30 multiple-choice questions in 30 minutes. Select a topic of similar difficulty that you haven't previously studied. Record the percentage of answers that are correct and compare the difference. The research indicates that the test-study-retest will beat the study-then test in most instances.

The benefit of taking these actions is that your study will stick.

## SUMMARY

Now you know that just reading and memorising is not the best method for retaining information, it's time to adopt a deliberate practice. Deliberate practice is more demanding mentally, but it gets results.

Consider your curriculum, work out the high-value topics (including ones you dislike!) and allocate appropriate testing time for these topics, preferably before you've studied them. Testing before studying will make a difference to your recognition memory and will help you retrieve the answers to objective questions.

You now know how to use your recognition memory. In the next chapter, you will be using your recall memory. The next chapter is all about being clear and concise on your key messages in your essay and short answer questions. You want to communicate in a way that the messages are understood.

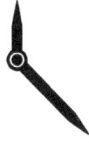

# CHAPTER SIX

# GET TO THE POINT

This chapter will build on the skills and knowledge from the last chapter to answer another form of common exam question, such as written short answer questions or essays. We initially discuss ways to improve your written communication. Then we will describe how you can develop an overview of the types of questions that come up regularly at every exam. With this knowledge, you can plan these answers, so you get to the point quickly with a message that is loud and clear. Then we will explain how you can increase your focus and decrease your fear of responding incorrectly by using a pre-performance routine. Using this pre-performance routine before reading each question also gets you in the zone, and you are more likely to be succinct and relevant in your responses. Lastly, we will give you a technique to link your handovers and work scenarios to the scenarios you are presented with for each clinical question in the exams. Again, this enables you to be more succinct in your responses to questions.

You have a wealth of information on most topics. When asked questions that test your recall, you must communicate that information succinctly in exams. Recognition and recall are different. Recognition requires you to choose a correct answer from other plausible choices. Recall requires you to communicate your answers to the exam questions in bullet points or prose.

Take a question such as this. *"Did Daniel Craig star as James Bond in No Time to Die"*? With recognition memory, you just answer 'yes' or 'no'. Whereas if the question was *"Who was the star of the James Bond movie, No Time to Die?"*, then you have to search your brain for cues. Think of other questions where you must use your recall memory. What cues do you use to nudge your memory? Write those cues down and see if you can work out the logical steps you took to remember these cues. Cues could be words, sentences, images, or incomplete pictures. As long as they have some connection to the information you are attempting to retrieve. Be aware of the differences between recall and recognition memory, so that your study will be appropriate for the exam components in your college exams.

The metaphor we use is that you train for the race you are running. So, if you are doing short answer questions then you practise for that and if you are doing essay answers, practise those.

The amount of time allocated for the exam may require that each short answer question be completed in four minutes, or perhaps 10 minutes, or 15 minutes, depending on the specialty. In some specialties, there are more extended essay questions. It may be necessary to complete these in 30 minutes, or perhaps one hour, depending on the time allowed for the exam. Time seems to be an essential factor in most recall exams – candidates are pushed to finish on time.

You will need to develop an overview of the material you need to recall and the topics that repeatedly appear in exams (we will show you how later in this chapter). The ability to provide correct responses to these questions is considered significant for your specialty. This is where you gain marks.

Once again, the key to this is testing and retesting. Factors you will get great at by testing and retesting exam questions to polish your answers are:

- the type of ideal answers you were given in study groups or tutorials
- the questions and answers that repeatedly come up each year in exams that involve short or long answers in your own words.

It might seem like a waste of time to test and retest when there is so much to learn, but over time you develop a feel for the types of questions asked. It is easier when you establish a template for answering questions.

One of the most significant barriers to getting this right is that being succinct takes courage. It's not that you don't know how to be succinct. You are succinct every day in your handover to other registrars. You use ISBAR for handovers (introduction, situation, background, assessment, referral, or recommendation). But when it comes to exams and sometimes handovers to intimidating consultants, it is all too easy to get flustered under pressure. It takes courage to communicate the answer succinctly. We will talk about the importance of being succinct in the next few paragraphs.

To be succinct, you must first give the overview or main message, then the key details, and then the supporting findings or evidence. You do so every day in your handover to other registrars. You can see this in the inverted pyramid in Chapter Seven of Leah Mether's 2019 book *Soft Is the New Hard*, where she talks about communication under pressure. The main part of the inverted pyramid is the message, the middle part consists of the details, and the pointy end of the pyramid consists of the evidence or findings. When registrars answer exam questions, they often try to second-guess the examiner. So, they write down everything related to the topic in their answers, hoping something will catch. This is the opposite of succinct. Using Mether's inverted pyramid – overview, then details, then findings – as a template for your answers will help you remain succinct. Even questions from left field can be answered with conviction and confidence using this template.

Most important and
newsworthy facts:
what's the story/your
message about?

The main story: what
are the key details?

Supporting content: what background or supporting evidence/
information will help persuade
and add weight to the argument?

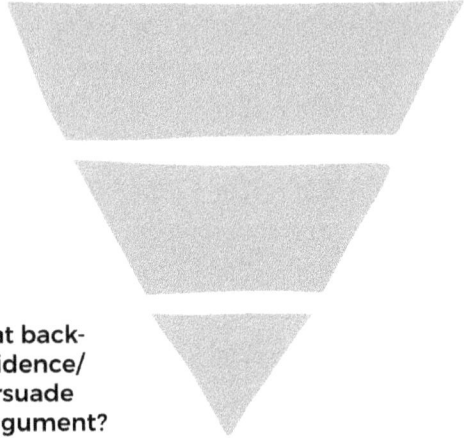

**Source:** Mether, Leah (2019) *Soft is the New Hard: How to Communicate Effectively Under Pressure*

In her book, Mether also talks about the message being able to pass the pub test, which is a helpful way to consider how you communicate. Imagine that a consultant fired a question at you, *"Can you tell me what's going on with that 57-year-old patient in Cubicle 2?"* As a junior doctor, you immediately launch into details. The consultant looks a little impatient at your long-winded answer. Now imagine that you went for a beer in the local pub that evening, and the patient's partner asked how his wife was getting on. In layperson's terms, you would give him an overview. In other words, you gave him a succinct message. Now, if you had answered the consultant with the same overview, albeit in professional terms, you would have given a succinct and clear message. That passes the pub test.

After written exams, colleges provide minimal feedback on the reasons for failure. However, one comment that is consistently made each year by almost every college is that the candidate did not answer the question being asked. When we talked to some of these candidates about their exam failures, they felt they had given a complete answer. When we probed a little deeper, they admitted that they were excited to get a particular question because:

- they read around the topic only the week before
- they wrote everything they knew about the topic in their answer
- they spent more time than was allocated on that question, which meant that they had less time on the remaining questions
- they were expecting to get top marks on that answer.

The problem was that, although the candidate might have had a wealth of information on that topic, they did not concisely communicate their answer to the question. Instead, they were too excited about having a topic they thought they knew well.

## KEIRA'S STORY

*Keira was doing her Fellowship intensive care exam in which her written exam consisted of two papers, each with 15 ten-minute short answer questions. Keira kept to the time on the morning paper. In the afternoon paper, to her joy, she saw that the tenth question was on a topic she had studied the previous week. This was a chance to get top marks. Keira went four minutes overtime on her answer because she had so much to write. It should have been completed in 10 minutes. In her excitement to communicate all she knew on the topic, she overlooked answering the specific question. She had to scramble to finish the last five questions before time was up. She only had time to put down a few points with that last question.*

*A few weeks later, Keira received her results. She had failed. She was advised she hadn't given the appropriate answer on the question where she had hoped to achieve the maximum marks. On three of the following five questions, she had received a fail mark because there wasn't enough information. Unfortunately, this happens all too often. A disappointed Keira learned a valuable lesson – keep to time and answer the relevant question.*

## What you can do right now to make a change

ASK A RANGE OF CONSULTANTS, SOME POSSIBLY PREVIOUS
EXAMINERS, TO MARK YOUR SHORT ANSWER QUESTIONS.

Many of your consultants are empathetic to exam candidates and
will go out of their way to help you. But often, the best feedback
is the critical feedback from the consultants about whom you are
apprehensive – have the courage to ask for genuine feedback
from a range of consultants and do your short answer questions
honestly, without reading around the topic first to create a "perfect
answer", however tempting that is!

The benefit of doing this is that, despite the possibility that you may
feel consultants will think less of you, because of your perceived
unsatisfactory answers, you will get critical and useful feedback
prior to actually sitting the exam.

## DEVELOP AN OVERVIEW OF STUDY TOPICS

What are the top value topics? What is this topic about? Get an overview
of the topics and types of questions that have been asked in exams in
previous years. Most colleges release these questions each year. In each
specialty, some topics are particularly important, and questions are always
asked on these topics at each exam.

> By taking the time to go through five to 10 years'
> worth of questions asked previously, you will see
> patterns emerging. Sometimes the same question
> comes up each year with different wording.

Be careful about going back any further than ten years as occasionally
medical techniques change.

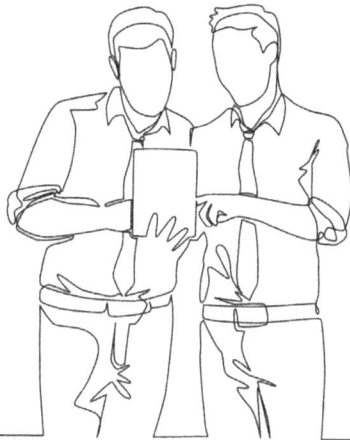

Spend an hour going through all the past papers and tallying the number of questions on each topic. You may be surprised at how often the same topics appear repeatedly. You can efficiently structure your study to focus on the important, frequently tested topics first and spend less time on the topics that appear only once or twice. Perhaps you'll notice how often the candidate is required to draw up a table to critically evaluate different methodologies. You will also know how many management or treatment questions come up. In this way, you will develop an understanding of what the examiners have been testing over the years. This enables you to select important topics for study where you feel your knowledge is not up to scratch. Focusing on what you don't know rather than what you already know builds confidence that you are tackling the right topics. When you know topics well, you dare to be more precise and concise in your responses to questions.

## ZITA'S STORY

*Zita had failed once before, about a year ago. When asked how often she studied for that exam, she indicated that she just snatched hours whenever she could. She didn't have any particular plan, and often felt overwhelmed by the amount of material she had to cover. However, a few months before her second attempt at the exam, Zita decided to become more organised. She spent a couple of hours meticulously writing up a spreadsheet that outlined the questions and topics that came up regularly in each exam over the previous eight years. Doing this helped Zita organise her study so that she studied and tested herself on topics of high value, where she felt her knowledge was deficient. In addition, writing up a spreadsheet and focusing primarily on the high-value material gave Zita more confidence to prepare well for the exam. She was thrilled to pass at her next attempt at the exam.*

## What you can do right now to make a change

REVIEW PREVIOUS EXAM QUESTIONS TO PLAN YOUR STUDY TOPICS

Develop a spreadsheet using between five and ten years' worth of questions. Most recall questions from previous exams are available online. For example, what are the high-value questions that come up each year? What are the esoteric questions that come up occasionally? How many "discuss and critically evaluate" questions come up each year? These are the hardest. How many "list, summarise, or outline" questions come up? These are easier to recall. Put a score out of 10 next to each of the questions in all the previous exams to ascertain what you think you already know or don't know.

The benefit of doing this is that any low score, particularly on the high-value topics, highlights where your knowledge is deficient and can guide you to choose which topics you should emphasise in your study.

## OVERCOME THE FEAR, USE PRE-PERFORMANCE ROUTINES

A pre-performance routine is any routine or habit that a performer, athlete, or professional does to enhance their performance, get into the right mindset, and combat anxiety. Elite athletes, particularly in individual sports such as gymnastics and diving, commonly use pre-performance routines to get in the zone before they perform. For example, they may have a ritualised warm-up, listen to the same music playlist, use the same positive affirmations, or take a set number of counted diaphragmatic breaths.

The pre-performance routine that we recommend for short answer questions and essays is:

1. Take a diaphragmatic breath before reading the scenario and question. It lowers the heart rate and focuses attention.
2. Underline the keywords in the scenario and the question. This emphasises their importance in your short-term memory.
3. Write headings. This will help you organise and structure your response.

This routine is helpful for written exams using booklets. If your exam is online, make sure you have paper at hand so you can write the keywords and/or headings to emphasise these before commencing your typed response.

This pre-performance routine helps bring you to your optimal performance zone. You now have your full attention on the question and your response. All external and internal distractions are minimised.

<blockquote>
Keeping yourself calm during your exam and having a routine to follow allows for sustained attention throughout the hours of the exam.
</blockquote>

If you have total focus on each question, you are more likely to be clear and concise in your message.

A pre-performance routine gives structure and a plan for each short answer, question, or essay. If you decide to use it, then you need to do it before every question in every mock exam, study group, or home testing from now on. With practice, taking time to do a pre-performance routine becomes automatic, which helps you focus more readily on the response.

Agnes Moors and Jan De Houwer, in their 2006 article "Automaticity: A Theoretical and Conceptual Analysis" in the *Psychological Bulletin*, discuss several theoretical views of automaticity. They suggest that automaticity allows you to perform tasks quickly, efficiently, and effortlessly after sufficient practice. Automaticity is the ability to do things without occupying the mind with the low-level details required, allowing it to become an automatic response pattern. Because the pre-performance routine is automatic, you won't panic on a question you don't know. If you are interrupted and need to refocus, redo your pre-performance routine. This automaticity before every written question reduces the energy required by your brain.

If you have a pre-performance routine for every question, you are more likely to think calmly and mindfully about a response. You control the fear and stay in the right mindset. When you come across a short answer or essay question that normally spikes the adrenaline and causes panic, you just automatically do your pre-performance routine and create positive behavioural changes. These behavioural changes include lowering the heart rate and reducing the fight or flight response.

According to Jean Williams in her 2010 book, *Applied Sport Psychology*, you can selectively attend to the cues of the task at hand while screening out irrelevant and distracting stimuli by reducing that fight or flight response. In addition, automatically incorporating a pre-performance routine before every written question minimises the chance of brain freeze or panic.

Patsy remembers an email from a grateful psychiatry registrar who finally passed his Fellowship exam. It was his last attempt, and he was having trouble with his essays. The pre-performance routine made such a difference for him. *"Your techniques were spot on and I followed everything you instructed me to do, right down to the routine on the day of the exam. Importantly, you helped me believe that I could pass the exam and just needed some tweaking with answers and help also with managing my anxiety around it."*

Did you know that the Australia and New Zealand College of Anaesthetists has a pre-performance routine for mixing drugs? They don't call it that, but that is what it is. Anaesthetists must check they prescribe the right drugs in the correct quantity to the right patient. They look at the labels, check the expiry date, even though a technician may previously have done that, make sure the drug in the ampoule is the right colour as the correct dose is transferred to the syringe, then label the syringe. The college insists on this routine for all anaesthetists when they mix and give drugs to patients to minimise any errors.

Imagine an anaesthetist driving into the hospital for a 7:30 am start. She only just avoids an accident with a large truck at an intersection. When she arrives at work, her adrenaline is still high, and she feels a little shaken. However, when mixing drugs for the first patient, she automatically evaluates each step as she gets ready. She's done it hundreds of times before. Her chances of making a mistake are minimised because of this pre-performance routine.

## What you can do right now to make a change
### USE DIAPHRAGMATIC BREATH TO RECOVER FROM DISTRACTIONS OR INTERRUPTIONS

During the exam, somebody having a coughing fit, a fire alarm going off, or a sudden announcement by the invigilator is an interruption. You need to have a strategy, such as a pre-performance routine, where you can refocus your attention back to the exam response. We suggest that you learn to take a diaphragmatic breath immediately after any distraction to the thought processes, whether you are at home or work. For example, you are reading a research paper during your allocated study time on your day off. Your partner is minding the baby. However, he keeps interrupting you to ask where to find items like clean nappies. If you take a big breath before answering your partner, it will keep the frustration out of your voice. Then take another big breath to refocus back onto the research paper.

The benefits of doing this are that you now have a way to control that fight or flight response. Do it often enough, and when a situation arises in an exam that is a distraction, you will automatically take a big breath and refocus your attention.

## BE AUTHENTIC! LINK WORK SCENARIOS TO EXAM SCENARIOS

Registrars tell us that they are often instructed by consultants to take responsibility for, or ownership of, a patient. They want you to do this in your everyday work situations, particularly when you hand over to the next shift's healthcare team. And of course, you endeavour to give the best of care to your patients during your work shifts. You also usually communicate succinctly when you hand over the care of your patients at the end of each shift. Therefore, it makes sense that many short answer and essay-type questions have clinical scenarios that attempt to mimic the information you have available before examining a patient in a work situation.

Consultants are aware that you behave differently in an exam, although you may be competent at work. You more than likely treat the exam as an ordeal, impacting how you answer the questions – you do not give succinct explanations or responses. The consultants want you to behave as you usually do in a work situation.

Instead of thinking of the exam fearfully as an enormous hurdle, think of it as a challenge. A challenge may be difficult and require intense focus and training, but it is approached with a confident (and even excited) mindset.

You have years of experience taking histories and examining patients. Why not mentally try to link any of these experiences to exam stems, the short scenarios you read before any questions in some exam components?

You can do this with the use of imagery. Create a mental picture of a patient with the relevant symptoms. When you do this in a written exam, your writing is more interesting, and you remember small details that indicate you have empathy towards the patient. The examiner who is marking your response will notice this. In an oral exam, the examiner will be more engaged with your answer. They listen to you and don't overlook any crucial points you may make. You pay more attention to your response rather than focusing on the examiner to ascertain whether you sound intelligent and professional and see if their face shows approval or otherwise.

By having a picture of a patient with similar symptoms in your mind, you sound, look, and feel more authentic. Your total attention is on your response. By paying more attention to your answer, rather than focusing on pleasing the examiner, you are less likely to miss details.

## WHAT'S THE EVIDENCE?

Paul Holmes and David Collins, in 2001, published an article, "The PETTLEP Approach to Motor Imagery: A Functional Equivalence Model for Sports Psychologists" in the *Journal of Applied Sport Psychology.* This imagery model provides a framework for the effective execution of imagery interventions. The model's abbreviation, PETTLEP, stands for the seven key components to consider when developing an intervention:

- physical
- environmental
- task
- timing
- learning

- emotion
- perspective.

The model is based on the notion that brain structures are activated during imagery, and if one thinks of the seven key components, this enhances the efficacy of the imagery. Thus, the imagery should be as realistic and as detailed as possible.

Imagine a lemon sitting on a plate in front of you. It is cut into slices with juice oozing out onto the plate. You are hot and thirsty. It looks so tempting. You pop a piece of lemon in your mouth and start chewing. Are you now salivating at the thought of chewing on a lemon? Probably! Most people salivate when they pretend they are chewing on a lemon. You are salivating because the brain sends messages down to the cells in the mouth to release saliva. The release of the saliva is meant to mitigate the stringent taste of the lemon juice. But you don't have a lemon in your mouth!

Now, you might imagine yourself at work on a busy morning on day shift, in your scrubs, and caring for your patient. You remember the ward environment, the sun streaming in through the windows, the nurses in their navy scrubs at the workstation, and the procedural task you were carrying out. You picture yourself with that patient – talking, smiling, asking questions, listening to answers, and being totally in the moment.

Your brain doesn't know when you pretend. If you pretend that the patient in the exam scenario is your patient or pretend that you are discussing your patient with another registrar, then what you write will be more authentic. This authenticity will engage the examiner when they read your answer to the question. They won't overlook any important points you may make. And because your brain believes that you are there, you will pay more attention to your response, and you are more likely to give a clear, relevant, and more concise answer to the short answer question or essay question.

# SUMMARY

There is a nearly infinite amount of study you can do in medicine – but the purpose of this study is to pass your exam, so concentrate on the high-value topics. Get an overview of exams over the years, so you can organise what topics to study most. Using a simple spreadsheet will focus your study time on the most important topics.

Then, every time you test yourself, do a pre-performance routine so that it becomes automatic. The pre-performance routine reduces your anxiety and makes "every day like the exam, and the exam like every day". If gold-medal Olympians use pre-performance routines to ensure peak performance in high-pressure situations, you can use them to control anxiety and before an exam.

The powerful imagery of putting yourself in your usual workspace, imagining you are using your skills to help one of your old patients, lends authenticity to your exam performance.

In the next chapter, we discuss non-verbal communication. Colleges usually run clinical exams several weeks and even months after the written exams. So instead of writing your answer, you need to verbally communicate those important findings succinctly and confidently. You'll learn a lot about yourself, and that can be fun.

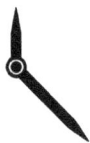

CHAPTER SEVEN

# NON-VERBAL COMMUNICATION UNDER PRESSURE

This chapter will start with an introduction to non-verbal communication in the workplace. Then we'll look at how to appear confident and calm to give a good impression when you first meet with the examiners. You need to develop an awareness of your body – your posture, facial expressions, and hands. We then talk about how to use your voice to communicate with understanding. Examiners make judgements on the way you sound. So, it is essential to be aware of how your voice sounds. Next is how to correct your presentations and interviews using self-feedback. And finally, we talk about imagery and how it can change perceptions and improve how you communicate.

Non-verbal communication is our body language and everything we communicate besides the spoken word – posture, use of physical space, gestures, clothing and appearance, facial expressions, and tone of voice. The non-verbal communication cues – the way you listen, look, move, and react – tell the person you're communicating with whether you care, if you're being authentic, and how well you're listening. Even the way you enter the exam room is an example of non-verbal communication – do you stride confidently, straight-backed, and take up space in the room, or do you slide in unobtrusively and stand at a distance? "Owning" your space projects confidence (and competence).

Paralanguage is known in linguistics as the non-verbal elements of speech used to modify meaning and convey emotion, such as pitch, speech rate, volume, and intonation. The way you speak amplifies or diminishes the content of your speech. If you mumble or speak in a soft monotone, it is not only boring and challenging for the examiner to understand, it also displays hesitancy and lack of confidence.

Verbal communication, non-verbal communication, and empathy play essential roles in patient–doctor and doctor–examiner encounters. Knowing what non-verbal communication involves improves your verbal communication, especially in clinical exams and interviews. The examiner's visual perception of your non-verbal communication affects their perception and interpretation of your verbal communication. What do you want examiners to experience when they meet you? Ideally, you want to demonstrate good posture, a pleasant and calm demeanour, and a confident and clear voice. Chapter Six talked about linking work scenarios to exam scenarios for the written short answer questions. The same applies in clinical vivas. Where possible, link your previous experiences at work with the exam scenarios you are given. This will make your verbal replies more authentic and engaging to the examiners.

Whether on a screen or face-to-face, your examiner is watching you as you respond to the question.

If can imagine that the examiner is just another registrar, you are more likely to remain calm, access the appropriate response in your memory, and give a confident and authentic answer. Your brain has been tricked again into believing that it's real!

Examiners are human. They get tired, bored, and lose attention. When candidates look calm and confident when they first meet them, the examiners relax. If a candidate seems nervous and edgy, they think, *"This is going to be hard work."* If examiners are impressed by a candidate's calm, confident demeanour, then a small error may be overlooked. If they already have the impression the candidate is unsure of themselves, that same small error may reinforce their first impression.

If you have poor non-verbal communication, the examiners will not engage easily with you. They might lose attention and ask more questions because they weren't listening closely, or they might question what you say (because you appear unsure of yourself). They might even miss important points because they tuned out from your monotonous presentation.

Remember when you were in med school and had new lecturers at the beginning of a semester? Within 20 to 25 seconds, you could tell whether you liked them or not. Of course, you didn't know why, and you might well have changed your mind later. However, if you liked the new lecturer, it affected how you reacted. It made a difference to how much you enjoyed the lecture and how focused you were on their presentation.

## APPEAR CONFIDENT AND CALM, NO MATTER WHAT

You want to be dynamic in your approach, particularly if you have cross-table vivas or the examiner is an observer as you engage with an actor who is pretending to be a patient. Use gestures, at least with one hand – don't sit frozen with a worried expression on your face, clenched teeth, and hunched shoulders. You want the examiner to be engaged. If they are engaged, they will watch you and listen intently to your answer. First, breathe and straighten your posture. Keep your body upright, straighten your shoulders, hold your head high, and keep your hands away from your face. Maintain good eye contact with the examiner (or the actor, if you have one). If you are one of those doctors who tries to gauge if the examiner is approving or disapproving of what you are saying, that could mean you don't trust your response. Don't get into the habit at work of answering based on whether you think the expression on the faces of your consultants is approving or disapproving. Examiners are often given instructions to appear bland and avoid giving feedback to the candidate through their non-verbal expressions. Some examiners are better than others at this! Do not let this put you off your answer.

A combination of open and closed body language keeps the examiner more engaged. For example, if you are in a closed position, you might have your arms folded, legs crossed, or be positioned at a slight angle from the person with whom you are interacting. On the other hand, in an open posture, you might be directly facing the person with hands apart on the arms of the chair. The proportions in which you use closed and open body language are key in how examiners perceive you and remember your message.

A good ratio is approximately 70% open body language and 30% closed body language. Using open body language means the examiner is more likely to perceive you and your message as open. For example, a straight body and a pleasant expression on your face give a favourable impression to the examiner.

To have a pleasant facial expression, you must first be aware of your face. Some people look grumpy when they think their face is relaxed. Patsy learned this the hard way. Over a few drinks, her graduate psychology students have often told her that they feared her in class. She was surprised. She thought she was a pussy cat! So, she decided to see what she looked like in the mirror while giving a lecture. Unbeknownst to her, her resting face did look a little grumpy! So she practised in the mirror what a "pleasant face" looked like and trained herself to use these facial muscles more consistently. Try it yourself. A pleasant resting face makes you and your examiner feel more comfortable and relaxed.

By appearing calm and confident, the examiner will perceive you that way. As a result, your examiner will listen to your responses with more attention. This may positively affect your marks as they will not inadvertently miss any statements you make. A better understanding of this type of communication may also lead to developing stronger relationships with colleagues and patients.

## JASON'S STORY, TOLD BY PATSY

*I recently consulted with a young doctor, Jason, who had initially failed to get into a competitive orthopaedic surgery program. He had already spent time and money learning to improve his content and came to me for the non-verbal communication component. I immediately became aware that his non-verbal communication was poor.*

*At first, I thought he was just shy, but it became a little frustrating after a while. Jason seldom looked me in the eye when talking. His face looked wooden, and he never smiled. He also didn't respond if I made a light-hearted comment. I asked him a question – one of the questions he'd been asked in the interview – and he gave a comprehensive answer, but his voice was monotone. He looked disinterested, his head was down, and he was not squarely facing me. I could see why he was not chosen for the training program. I realised that we had a lot of work to do.*

*Over the next few months, Jason made significant changes in many aspects of his non-verbal communication. Understandably, Jason felt at first that the changes were artificial, like acting a part. He said, "It's not me, it's not how I am." However, he persisted and became more comfortable with the changes. I had persuaded him that he would be giving himself a much better chance of getting onto the program at his next interview. Sure enough, he was successful in his second attempt.*

Regular reminders can help to change old habits into new ones. We recommend using an interval timer. This is a device designed to assist athletes with the timing of interval workouts. We use a specific one called Gymboss (available online) that can be placed under your clothes at the start of the day. You can keep on using it even when in theatre, as it is under your scrubs. The Gymboss can be set to make a sound or vibrate against your skin at regular intervals throughout the day. This is a valuable reminder for various techniques, such as taking a diaphragmatic breath, straightening your posture, or increasing the volume of your voice.

## What you can do right now to make a change

### USE A NEUROHACK

If you want to use the interval timer to remind you to use a technique, think up a neurohack. A neurohack is a shortcut for cognitive processes. Let's say you want to improve your posture when you feel that vibration of the interval timer. In our practice, the neurohack we use for this is "thumbtack", that little pin that you push into a notice board. Using this word is effective in straightening the body and pushing the shoulders back. So when you become aware of the vibration of the interval timer, just imagine a thumbtack being pushed between your shoulder blades. At the same time, why not take that diaphragmatic breath to lower the heart rate.

The benefit is that you will, with regular practice, be perceived as more confident and calmer — and you will feel that way as well.

Here's another activity demonstrating how posture can have positive or negative effects. Choose to sit in one of two positions. One position is to sit big with legs outstretched and arms across the back of a chair or behind your head to make yourself big. The other position is to sit small by slumping, sitting on your hands, crossing your knees, and making yourself very small. Whichever position you choose, stay that way for a few minutes.

Then imagine standing up and presenting a patient's history to many consultants from various departments. Reflect on how you felt at the thought of standing up and presenting to this group. Did the position you chose, either big or small, make any difference to you?

The big position may make you feel more confident as there is a slight increase in testosterone. On the other hand, the small position may make you feel more nervous due to a slight increase in cortisol. The effects can be subtle, but the benefit is that you may become aware of how you feel at the thought of standing up in front of all those consultants. Is it different from what you would typically feel when presenting a patient's history to another registrar?

Dana Carney, Amy Cuddy, and Andy Yap presented research in 2010 on the embodied effects of expansive (vs contractive) non-verbal displays. They indicated that a large pose would lead to increases in testosterone, and a small pose would lead to increases in cortisol. The results are now considered to be inconclusive, based on Kristopher Smith and Coren Apicella's 2017 paper "Winners, Losers, and Posers: The Effect of Power Poses on Testosterone and Risk-taking Following Competition." But why not try to maintain a confident posture when under pressure? You have nothing to lose. And it may well work for you.

## BETTER COMMUNICATION USING THE VOICE

At the beginning of this chapter, we mentioned paralanguage – the non-verbal elements of speech used to modify meaning and convey emotion, such as pitch, volume, and intonation. People judge others by how they speak – how the words sound, not just what they say.

Voices are flexible. You can speak with passion, with authority, with humour. Your voice can convey warm concern, disinterest, or contempt; you can inspire or soothe just with your tone. But often, your voice, either when being evaluated or when speaking in public, becomes restricted, quiet, and monotonous because of nerves and muscle tightening. The skill of public speaking is to take control over how your audience perceives your voice. You want to sound interested and enthusiastic about the topic. There are several elements you need to be aware of and control to do this.

Five main elements will improve your communication skills under pressure:

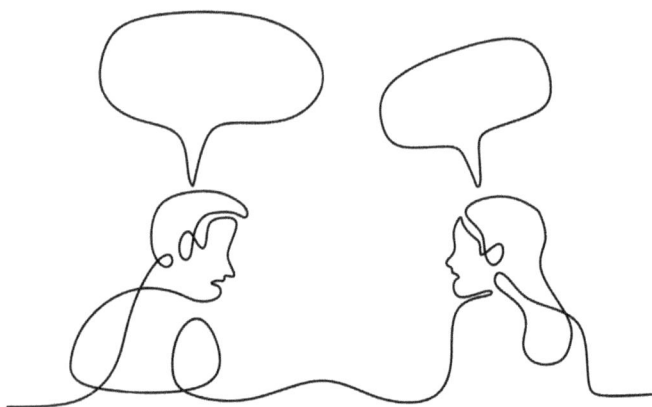

1. **Volume.** The diaphragm produces this. You are perceived as having competence, authority, and confidence. The use of your breath helps increase the magnitude of the voice.
2. **Pitch.** When talking, this is the range of the voice, the highs, and the lows. For example, we all know that lowering your voice at the end of a sentence denotes a full stop, whereas finishing a sentence on a high note indicates a question. And if someone constantly talks in a monotone, it's not long before we lose interest.
3. **Resonance or tone.** This involves the soft palate and sinuses. This is the difference between speaking with a nasal twang or an open

throat. Resonance is associated with authority and influence. Radio announcers must rely on their voice to project conviction, whereas the occasional sports announcer on TV seems to place trust in their good looks.

4. **Diction.** This involves fine control over the small muscles around the mouth, lips, and tongue, enunciating each syllable of every word to provide clarity. If English is your second language and you have a strong accent but practise good diction, it is easier to comprehend what is being said.

5. **Pace and pause.** Speaking slowly allows your listener to engage with the content of your speech and gives them time to reflect and think. Pausing at the end of sentences improves your listener's comprehension. Not only that, but we've also discovered that doctors who speak too fast or have strong accents seem to slow down considerably when they focus on good diction. This makes it easier to understand what they are saying.

We've all been cornered by someone at a party where we are trying to get away. The person is monotonous, they talk without a pause, and you are no longer listening. It can be excruciating. You want your examiners or consultants to be engaged and listen intently to your responses. You won't get marks if the examiner can't hear you. And you won't get marks if you are so dull that they don't pay attention.

## ALETTA'S STORY, TOLD BY PATSY

*A young consultant, Aletta, had passed her Fellowship exams a couple of years previously and had just started a new job as a staff consultant at a small regional hospital. She felt awkward in her new job. She was the only female consultant in her department. She came to see us because she thought she wasn't being listened to. This seemed to be mostly whenever three or four consultants would have a quick impromptu meeting in the corridor or tearoom.*

*After talking to Aletta for a short time, I could understand why she wasn't being listened to. She was short, and most of the other consultants (male) were taller than her. Also, her voice, although well-modulated, was soft. She described how she kept her head down and seemed to have difficulty maintaining eye contact. We worked on three aspects of non-verbal communication:*

1. *posture to increase the perception of confidence*
2. *voice to increase the volume*
3. *eye contact as she spoke.*

*Better posture and eye contact were easy to change for Aletta. But she was reluctant to raise the volume of her voice. Her parents taught her when she was a child that raising her voice was unbecoming. I even stood her at the front door, and she had to converse with me at the other end of the hallway, a good four metres away. She felt she was shouting. I assured her she wasn't. Finally, with practice and a lot of laughs in the process, she managed to increase the volume of her voice. I received an email from Aletta a couple of weeks later. "The other consultants are listening to me now. Speaking up was the best thing I've done. I feel I'm now being respected a lot more. Thank you so much. It has made such a difference."*

## What you can do right now to make a change

### EXPLORE HOW VOCAL ELEMENTS CAN CHANGE MEANING

*"I didn't eat your lunch."* Here is a fun little exercise to demonstrate how this sentence can have several entirely different meanings. Grab a colleague, your partner, or a study buddy. Or, if you want to do it alone, record your answers on your phone and listen to them later. Person A says the sentence, *"I didn't eat your lunch,"* to person B, emphasising the first word. Now swap over, and person B says the sentence, *"I didn't eat your lunch,"* emphasising the second word.

Continue swapping over and moving the emphasis to the third, the fourth, and then the fifth word.

Notice how the sentence has an entirely different meaning, depending on which word is emphasised. This exercise invokes the vocal elements of pitch, volume, resonance, diction, pace, and pause.

If you want to highlight what you mean in each of the above messages even more, then repeat and incorporate the body language tips mentioned earlier as you emphasise each word of the sentence.

The benefit you derive from this exercise is that you become aware of how messages change their meaning, depending on how you emphasise certain words.

## SEEK FEEDBACK BECAUSE IT WORKS

We often think we are being clear, concise, and accurate in our content. We think we are conveying our message in a pleasant or interesting manner. It's not until we listen to our voices that we understand why we are not as clear and concise as we thought we were. You can obtain regular feedback regarding what you say and how you say it. Record your responses to verbal questions when under pressure and listen twice. The first time listen just to the content. Did you say everything you wanted to say? Did you omit anything? Then listen again, focusing just on the tone of voice. Do you sound tentative? Or do you sound confident and succinct?

This self-feedback is also helpful for interview practice. All doctors must interview to get onto accredited training programs, and later, you will need to interview for consultant positions. Self feedback is a tremendous learning tool. You'll soon learn to recognise when you sound confident and concise and when you sound doubtful and tentative, and you now have the tools to analyse why your voice sounds this way and which voice elements you need to adjust.

It is beneficial to record feedback from your consultants (with their permission) to listen to later. Consultants will primarily give feedback on your content but also ask them to give you specific feedback on your presentation as a whole – verbal and non-verbal. Listen to your recorded answer and the consultant's feedback when you get home. This reinforces what the consultant said and enables you to evaluate your content and re-organise your answers to improve clarity and brevity. However, always listen a second time to your recorded response. This is the double-take feedback method, where you listen only to the tone of your voice. The tone of voice indicates where you are tentative, where your voice sounds tense or unsure, and where you are confident and sure of your explanation. These are your "tells" – your verbal indicators that you lack confidence in the topic.

It is not the sort of feedback you would expect from consultants. You usually know where and why you feel flustered because you're unsure of the answer. Listening to it the second time can dredge up the negative feelings you experienced as you struggled with your response. Listening to your voice is hard. You will cringe at first, and you'll probably try to find excuses not to listen to the tone of voice. It doesn't sound the way you expect. Listening to your voice leads to a lack of objectivity. We strongly suggest that you pretend you are listening to a colleague on the phone. This distances you from your voice and enables you to be more objective and critical of how the voice sounds.

If you pretend you are listening to a colleague, you are better able to critique the voice if you ask three questions:

1. Do I like the voice?
2. Does it engage me?
3. Do I believe it?

If the recorded voice sounds doubtful, it encourages you to read around that specific topic later to ensure that you understand it. Sometimes the content is correct, but you are anxious in front of the consultant and scared of being wrong. This may make your voice sound tentative. You then recognise that you must believe in yourself and have the courage to speak up convincingly. You'll soon realise how your voice changes when you are flustered.

You'll also likely recognise that you don't have full attention to your response. First, this may be because you are focusing on the consultant's face for any sign of approval or disapproval. (Hint: To avoid seeing the consultant's micro-expressions, focus on the space between the eyes rather than in their eyes.) Second, with critical self-feedback, you can learn to ignore that inclination to listen to your words in an endeavour to impress the consultant. You want your focus to be entirely on your response. So, what feedback do you want to notice? Perhaps whether the volume of your voice has lowered, or you sound more tentative or waffly. Maybe you sit on the fence and give details first before an overview.

> With that knowledge you gain from self-feedback, your responses to questions will improve considerably.

Over time, you will become far more relaxed about listening to yourself, and the responses will be more articulate and concise.

## ALI'S STORY, TOLD BY KELL

*Ali was an international medical graduate trying to get onto an accredited specialty training program for the second time. Her consultants told her that she needed to be more confident, and her voice was too soft. At the beginning of our session, I asked Ali what a typical question would be and pretended that this was the interview. She recorded her response onto her phone, and I then gave her feedback. Although her answer was technically correct, it had no structure. She* had no introductory sentence and no conclusion. Her voice was soft and monotonous.

To help Ali structure her answer, I gave her an unusual analogy she found amusing – and helpful! It was a drawing of a filleted fish, with the head, the spine, the ribs, and the tail. The head represents an introduction, the spine represents the main flow of the story, and the ribs are the subtopics (or details). After every subtopic, Ali needed to return to the spine to continue answering the question. And when she had finished answering the question, the tail was the conclusion to let her listeners know she had ended her response.

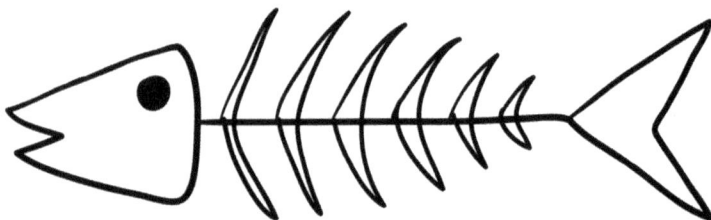

At the end of the session, I asked Ali to respond to the same question asked initially, and she was to re-record herself. Ali had embraced our comments during the consultation, particularly the analogy, which resonated with her. Her second recording was so much better. Her voice was louder, and she looked and sounded more confident. Her response to the question was clearer and more concise.

Later, Ali emailed us after listening to the two recordings at home. She was surprised and pleased that the second recording had improved so much. It convinced her that self-recording was a helpful exercise. She was using the double-take feedback method with success. A few weeks later, I was delighted to hear that she had been accepted onto the accredited training program of her choice.

# What you can do right now to make a change

## USE THE DOUBLE-TAKE FEEDBACK METHOD

When a consultant wants to ask a few questions, ask if you can record the responses and feedback. Later, after work, listen critically to your answers to the questions. First, listen just to the content for accuracy and any omissions. Compare it with the consultant's comments and then allocate a score out of 10 for the accuracy of the content. Then listen again to your response, but only to the tone of voice. You know you hate listening to your voice, so pretend you are listening to a colleague on the phone. Ask yourself those three questions mentioned above. Give yourself a score out of 10 for the tone of voice.

If you have any low scores, either for content or for any of the five voice elements, that means you should read around that topic again. What's missing? How could that response improve? You need to change one element at a time. Don't read around that topic that night, however. Instead, wait until your next study session when you can absorb the material into long-term memory. Then, a few days later, after the material is no longer in working memory, retest yourself on that question and note the improvement.

The benefit is that, with repetition, your responses to questions under pressure become more assured.

# IMAGERY CAN WORK WONDERS

Imagery is powerful, and you can use it to enhance your answers to verbal questions from examiners. Consciously exercising the direction of your imagery is a hallmark of mastery in sports, medicine, and any other areas of your life. Imagery combined with rich emotional texture effectively enhances perception and performance, no matter the situation. It can improve your performance in interviews and clinical exams, whether on a virtual screen or in person.

Clinical exam components are in different specialties such as surgery, emergency medicine, radiology, anaesthesia, critical care, basic physician training, and general practice. Exams may consist of objective structured clinical exams (OSCEs), short cases (Spots), cross-table vivas, describing images on the computer, history taking and examination of patients or actors, and possible later presentation of these in long and short cases. In the previous chapter, we mentioned that the brain could not distinguish between reality and imagination. However, the brain is remarkably clever at knitting together information, generating coherence, and filling in information. Therefore, if you can imagine a patient with similar symptoms to the question you've just been asked, the chances are that you'll sound authentic and empathic – and your attention will be firmly focused on your response.

Judy was sitting her clinicals for the second time. She was a basic physician trainee, and she had two long cases and four short cases across two separate exams. Judy felt confident about her long cases. They're typical of the length of time one takes to do a thorough examination. But like most basic physician trainees, Judy disliked the short cases. They are an exam-specific format that doesn't translate to real clinical practice. She worried she would not be able to get enough information in the seven minutes allowed for examination of the patient. In presenting findings to the examiner in the first attempt at the exam, she was flustered and stumbled over her words. In one case, she omitted to mention an important differential, even though she knew it.

## JUDY'S STORY, TOLD BY PATSY

*Judy was desperately anxious to pass. She and her partner wanted to start a family and didn't want to wait much longer. However, Judy's sabotaging thoughts increased the closer she got to the exam. She wondered if she should take beta-blockers to calm herself down in the short cases.*

*I gave her a different perspective. Indeed, not all interactions with patients were as extensive as in the long cases. After all, hospitals are busy places, and there are interruptions to lengthy examinations. Judy thought for a while and then remembered that she used to be involved with a patients' clinic once a week. There were always many people waiting in these clinics, and sessions tended to be short. I asked her to describe a situation that could easily be a short case in an exam. She recalled how she dealt with a previous patient in the clinic who may have had one or two similar symptoms. As she responded to that short case example, she pretended that it was her patient she was examining.*

*This resonated with her. She now saw the exam as a challenge rather than an ordeal. It changed her attitude from one of defeat to determination. She pictured examining or taking histories from patients in short cases in much the same way and for the same length of time that she would question patients in a clinic. As a result, Judy now sounds more authentic, acting more confidently, and I am confident that she will pass.*

You may have a mock exam that requires standing outside the room and reading a stem for two minutes. Let's say it's about a 57-year-old woman, Mrs Jones, who has pain in her abdomen. You search in your memory for a female you have previously treated, around the same age, who may have had the same initial complaint. In this way, by linking a real patient with the patient described in the stem, you are more likely to recall the questions that need to be asked to elicit the correct findings. What was your primary diagnosis? What other diagnoses were you considering? How did you refine your primary diagnosis and structure your differentials? By linking these work scenarios to possible exam scenarios, you will be more confident and empathic when talking to the examiner.

## SUMMARY

You have now learned how helpful non-verbal communication can be. Of course, you need to know the material for your clinical exams, but you also need to present it calmly and confidently. If you put in the effort to consciously adjust and optimise your non-verbal communication until it becomes a habit, you and others will notice the difference.

Perhaps focus on one or two of your voice elements that the double-take feedback method has highlighted need attention. Practise keeping your shoulders back (think thumbtack) and looking and sounding confident when responding to questions. Every time a consultant asks a question in a tutorial or mock exam, take a deep breath, adjust your posture before responding, and reply in a confident, loud voice.

In the next chapter we will talk about failure. Doctors don't learn how to fail in med school. When they fail their specialty exams, it hurts badly. We'll show you how to understand and rebound from failure, just like athletes – who fail more than they win.

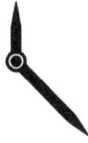

# CHAPTER EIGHT

# THE F WORD – LET'S TALK ABOUT FAILURE

Doctors often arrive at medical school with no experience of academic failure. As a group, you are more goal-oriented, driven, competitive, and perfectionistic than your non-medical peers. Although medical school is challenging, it has a very high pass rate, and many doctors start their specialist training in their late 20s or 30s, having never failed an exam. Until now.

Being a doctor does not make you immune to failure and error. On the contrary, being a doctor is a complex business with thousands of diseases to treat and many drugs and surgical procedures to choose from. As a result, trainee doctors often work at the edge of their capacity and competency, and they need to be resilient in the face of challenges, setbacks, and failures. At the same time, the rigorous exams that trainee doctors go through – with national pass rates of 70% – meaning that failure and setbacks are common. This outcome is challenging for doctors who appear infallible to the outside world.

In this chapter we will look at three strategies to help you manage failure. First we'll show you how approaching a challenge with a growth mindset can support your resilience and your ability to accept criticism and setbacks. Then we'll look at the thorny issue of blame, and the power of attribution. Finally, we'll talk about getting out of the rut of failure with adaptive coping strategies.

But before that, we would like you to take a moment to reframe your view of failure.

Failure is not the opposite of success; it's part of it. Success is often viewed as accomplishing an aim or purpose, while failure is considered the absence of success. These views imply that failure impedes success, which is inaccurate. While success is often thought of as a linear process (like the picture on the left), it's more like the picture on the right.

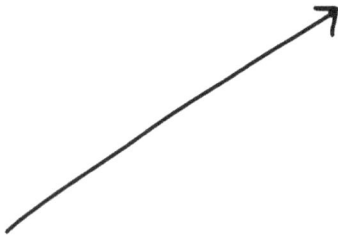

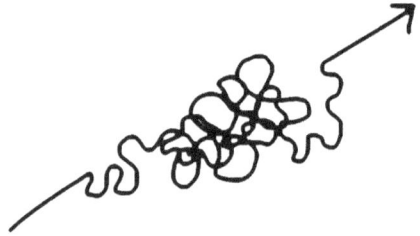

This concept of failure and setbacks as essential elements for success was shown in the 1997 Nike commercial that depicted the National Basketball Association's biggest star as a failure. In the ad, Michael Jordan recounted, that he had missed more than 9,000 shots in his career and had lost nearly 300 games and that he had been entrusted to take the game-winning shot

26 times and missed, and that because he failed over and over, that is why he has succeeded to become the best basketballer of all time. Going back further, when inventor Thomas Edison was working on the invention of the light bulb, his team was conducting a series of unsuccessful experiments. After making 1,000 unsuccessful attempts at inventing the lightbulb, a reporter asked, *"How did it feel to fail 1,000 times?"* Edison countered by saying, *"I have not failed. I've just found 1,000 ways that won't work."*

Don't get us wrong; failure feels like one of the worst things in life. Doctors who fail their exams often come to us feeling embarrassed, angry, guilt-ridden, or shamed. It's no wonder that we avoid failure. But failure is also a part of life. If you have ever watched children learn to walk, they fail a dozen times and get up again before succeeding. Failure and setbacks are necessary for their learning and continue to be necessary for our physical, emotional and intellectual growth throughout our lives.

While failure is a common element of being human, in the medical profession, failure is rarely discussed. Because of the implications for patient safety and a doctor's career, failure is seen as an aberrancy rather than an opportunity to learn and grow. But when approached correctly, medical errors offer you a chance to debrief what went wrong, learn, grow, build resilience, and change your response in the face of error.

Little attention is given to how trainee doctors can deal with failure in high-stakes exams. How you approach and manage failure impacts your resilience, growth, and wellbeing.

## APPROACHING A CHALLENGE WITH A GROWTH MINDSET

Let's start by considering the research on mindset by Stanford psychologist Carol Dweck. In her 2007 book, *Mindset*, she defines a fixed mindset as the belief that intelligence or ability is fixed and unchangeable. For example, some people are good at maths or art, or in medicine, some might have good analytical skills or be good communicators. In contrast, a growth mindset is a belief that intelligence or ability is malleable and that, through practice, you can improve.

The type of mindset that you have influences your desire to take on challenges and your ability to respond to failure. The mindset you have is influenced by the praise you received from your primary caregivers when you were young. In our practice, our clients often tell us that they would praise their children with words such as, *"You are so clever,"* or *"You are a natural at this."* This type of praise, although well-intentioned, promotes a fixed mindset.

Consider the praise you or others in your cohort might have received during school. Before entering your first medical lecture, you've likely been at the top of your class at school. When you attend your first medical lecture, all these students have been top performers throughout their school and academic career; now, there is a 50% chance of being below average. For the fixed mindset student, this can be difficult to deal with and affect the core of their being. This fixed mindset approach influences junior doctors who may shy away or not persist in the face of challenges or become highly anxious before exams.

In our practice, we often see people who have significant challenges with their studies and/or have failed their exams. Those doctors who have a growth mindset, as opposed to a fixed mindset, can better cope with the challenges or setbacks.

For example, let's look at a particularly challenging time growing up for many – the transition from primary school to high school. The environment is new, and often it involves lots of testing and new people. Around this time, students may disengage from learning. In a study published in *Child Development* by Carol Dweck and colleagues, titled "Implicit Theories

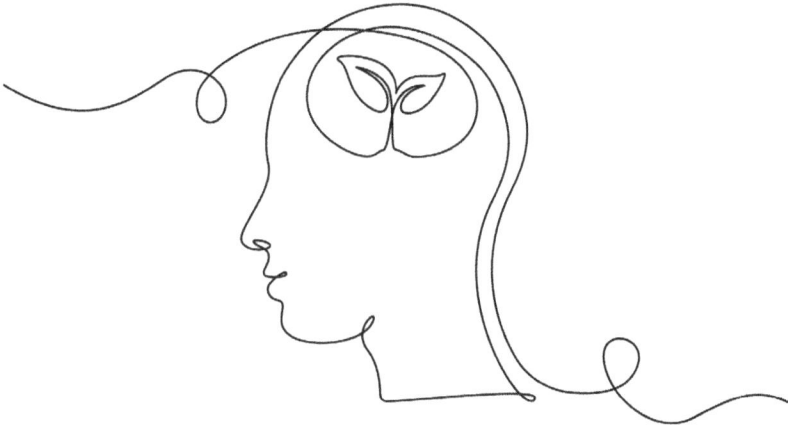

of Intelligence Predict Achievement Across an Adolescent Transition: A Longitudinal Study and an Intervention", it was found that students with a growth mindset in that transition period diverged well above those with a fixed mindset. According to Carol Dweck and the researchers, those with a growth mindset were more engaged and learned more, while those with a fixed mindset were disengaged in the face of challenges. Similar results have been displayed across various groups who have experienced difficult transitions, such as pre-med courses, sport, and the business world.

Mindset is crucial to perseverance and coping skills in the face of challenges and setbacks. The vignettes below are some typical examples that we see in our practice. These vignettes are fictional and based on our experiences. See if you can tell who has a fixed mindset and who has a growth mindset.

## DIFFERENT APPROACHES TO CHALLENGES AND FAILURE

### Vignette 1: Chiama
*Chiama was in an accredited program for anaesthetics. Yet, she kept on putting off sitting her primary exam. When asked why, she would say it was because she was "just not a problem-solving type of person." Her supervisor eventually lost patience and insisted she sign up for the*

*next sitting of the exam in four months. Reluctantly, she sat the exam and failed the written section, both the multiple-choice questions and the short answer questions. Chiama told her colleagues and friends that she was not surprised she did poorly. She was a bit off on the day of the exam.*

*She attended the first tutorial sessions for the next sitting, but after the consultant pointed out flaws in her logical reasoning and suggested some changes to her study methods, Chiama decided the consultant was intimidating her. She didn't attend any more tutorials and thought: "It is not my fault if I fail. Everybody is pushing me to sit this exam when I'm not ready." Chiama sat for the second time. She failed again and decided to drop out of the anaesthetics program.*

## Vignette 2: Mohammed

*Mohammed was excited to start working as an unaccredited junior registrar in a small unit in a private hospital. He knew he would have a lot to learn and knew that practical experience was the best way to gain the skills needed to eventually be a consultant. He was keen to learn from his senior colleagues. However, Mohammed wasn't prepared to be working so many night shifts with little variation in the presenting patient problems, and with little supervision or training because he was working overnight. He was disappointed but tried to think of the experience as an opportunity to learn, grow, and become a better doctor. Mohammed knew that he would eventually succeed if he put in the effort. He did extra shifts on his days off, at times when he was able to obtain constructive feedback from consultants. He learned many new procedures. The extra work and study paid off. Eventually, Mohammed was rotated to a larger teaching hospital and felt the thrill of being part of an effective medical team.*

## Vignette 3: Salek

*Salek was at the top of his class when he finished Year 12. He had always enjoyed school, and academic success had always come easily.*

*He was admitted to the school of medicine of his choice, and he was excited to prove his talent. But med school was different than expected, and when midterms were over, Salek was shocked to find that he had Cs in most of his subjects. Salek scheduled meetings with all his professors, and several of them suggested different ways to change his approach to notetaking and studying the course material. But Salek was confused by that. He knew he was smart, and smart kids don't have to study. If he must start studying now that he's in med school, does that mean he's not smart? Salek began to believe that he couldn't grasp the material. That made him anxious and upset. So, he became distracted by negative thoughts whenever he sat down to study. Most of his study time was spent worrying and thinking, "I have to do well on this next exam. I must get top marks. I'll never become a top surgeon if I don't get the best marks. Everyone is naturally smart. If I can't get top marks, maybe I'm just not good enough. Gee, what will people think of me?"*

Chiama (Vignette 1) and Salek (Vignette 3) have fixed mindsets. Chiama is *"just not a problem-solving type of person"*, and Salek *"knew he was smart, and smart kids don't have to study"*. Both Chiama and Salek believed those constructs to be unchangeable. However, in Vignette 2, Mohammed knew he would have a lot to learn and that, over time, he would improve his skills to eventually become a consultant with much effort. Mohammed demonstrates a growth mindset.

Mindset influences your desire to take on and persist through challenges. It also affects how you respond to feedback on how to improve and how you cope with failure. A person with a fixed mindset is likely to avoid challenges and become defensive in the face of feedback. We see this in Vignette 1 with Chiama avoiding the exam for as long as possible. She became defensive towards constructive feedback on improving her study skills and eventually dropped out of anaesthetics.

For the person with a fixed mindset, success is more about avoiding failure. Doctors with a fixed mindset see an academic challenge, like an exam, as a threat, with failure revealing a lack of intelligence or talent. They believe that exam success stems only from innate ability. For example, in Vignette 3, Salek believes "that he could not grasp the material", which profoundly affected his stress levels and self-esteem. Salek begins to question his self-worth. "If I can't get top marks, maybe I'm just not good enough."

On the other hand, a person with a growth mindset is likely to see learning as an opportunity to learn and seek out such challenges.

For example, in Vignette 2, Mohammed, while disappointed, tries to "think of the experience as an opportunity to learn, grow, and become a better doctor". As such, Mohammed is more optimistic that his efforts have agency, and he has greater perseverance in the face of challenges and setbacks than those with a fixed mindset.

Mindset influences your desire to take on challenges and your ability to persist through the challenge and respond to failure. A growth mindset influences your perseverance, resilience, and wellbeing. The type of mindset you have has significant implications on how you cope with setbacks and learn new skills. In Chapter Four, we talked about some common thinking traps. A fixed or growth mindset is the filter through which you view your experiences, and it changes your thought patterns.

To err is to be human. Everyone fails. JK Rowling had to overcome numerous rejections of her *Harry Potter* books. Steve Jobs was kicked out of Apple before leading Apple 10 years later. Failure rates across the nine main medical colleges in Australia range from 30% to 53%, according to their statistics, which are published annually. If you look at a study conducted by Westbrook and colleagues in 2010 in two major teaching hospitals in New South Wales, 9% of medication administrations were associated with the clinical error. This excludes timing errors.

## What you can do right now to make a change

ADOPT THE *YET* SOLUTION

This exercise is called the *yet* solution. This is a powerful three-letter word. According to Carol Dweck, we are all on a learning journey, and just because you might not have achieved what you were trying for does not mean that you should not try or that you should just give up. All it means is that you have not succeeded *yet* and that the pathway to future success is practice.

For example, if after an unsuccessful attempt you say to yourself, *"I'm not good at this,"* that can become, *"I'm not good at this yet." "I can't do it,"* becomes *"I can't do it yet."* Carol Dweck's research teaches children that the *yet* solution increases confidence and persistence. The power of *yet* is that it builds a bridge between having a fixed mindset and having a growth mindset.

What do you say to yourself after a failure or an unsuccessful attempt? Common fixed mindset examples are, *"If I can't do this, I'll be a failure,"* or *"If I had talent, I would've been able to do that."* Ask yourself if there is a growth mindset approach that you can use to counter this fixed mindset talk? For example, *"If I can't do this…"* could become, *"I might not be able to do this yet, but it's just going to take some practice."*

Often you can hold different mindsets about different topics such as maths and English. Mindsets can also change within a topic if you experience a trigger, such as feedback or a high-pressure exam. It's important to:

- know the triggers that push you into a fixed mindset, and

- develop a *yet* solution that creates a bridge from the fixed to the growth mindset.

For example, in our practice, we had a junior doctor who had mostly a growth mindset but noticed that when his supervisor made constructive/critical comments on a particular procedure, he would switch into a fixed mindset in the face of specific criticism. This was having an impact on his stress, anxiety, and overall wellbeing. We identified what he was saying to himself in this trigger situation. It was *"I am hopeless and can't do this"*. We asked him to change those thoughts to *"I might not be able to do this yet, and I am learning each day as I practise more."*

In other words, your *yet* is coming; your *yet* is not yet here.

For some people, the *yet* solution does not resonate. However, slightly changing a statement can make a big difference in a person adopting a growth mindset. For example, you might have a common fixed mindset of *"It's too hard,"* which can be transformed into a growth mindset phrase of, *"I'll keep trying." "I can't do that"* could be changed to a growth phrase of *"How can I get better at that?"*

## WHO IS TO BLAME?

In our experience, doctors who fail their exams often begin with questions such as *"Why did this happen?" "What did I do wrong?" "What could have been done differently?"* In short, they do an attributional search for the causes of their failure. In our work with doctors, this attributional search falls into three broad themes that influence how the doctors respond to their failure.

1.  **Responsibility.** This theme asks whether the cause was initiated from them (for example, I was responsible) or outside of them (someone else was responsible). For example, we worked with John, who failed his exam because he attributed his failure to a lack of ability. John had an *internal* locus of control. Another candidate, Archie, failed his medical exam, and he attributed his failure to both an unfair exam and that he was using subpar study resources. Archie had an *external* locus of control.

2.  **Stability.** Here doctors often ask the likely probability of the cause changing over time – is it permanent or not permanent across time and situations? John, mentioned above, attributed his failure to a lack of ability, which is stable because it's unlikely to change. We were also working with another client, Mary, who failed her exam and attributed this to being sick and exhausted. In this case, Mary might attribute this failure to being unstable as illness and fatigue are temporary factors, so her response to failure is likely to be more resilient than John's response. John's internal and stable attribution is likely to lead to low morale and lower expectations for the future. This dimension elicits feelings of hopelessness.

3.  **Controllability.** In this theme, doctors either attribute the cause of failure as within their control, such as their skills, or they view it as outside of their control (such as luck or others' actions). For example, Mustafa, a client of ours, failed his exam because he did not study efficiently and effectively. In this case, the cause is controllable because Mustafa could have studied differently. However, other clients attributed their failure to a lack of ability, such as John, above. In those cases, the cause is uncontrollable. Attributing failure due to controllable factors, such as effort, elicits feelings of guilt and regret. On the other hand, attributing failure to a lack of ability or aptitude, which is not controllable, evokes feelings of humiliation and shame, involving social comparisons with others who might have passed the exam.

According to Bernard Weiner and colleagues in their book *Perceiving the Causes of Success and Failure*, the different combinations of these three themes result in four common attributions to success and failure that we see all the time with junior doctors. Below is a table of the different attributions that we see doctors make when they fail their exams and what they typically say to themselves. Each of these four ways doctors attribute failure influences their self-esteem and how they will view past failures and future challenges.

| ABILITY:<br>internal, stable, uncontrollable | TASK DIFFICULTY:<br>external, stable, uncontrollable |
|---|---|
| e.g. I am not smart enough to understand the questions in the exam. Therefore, I will never become a successful doctor. | e.g. The questions were impossibly hard. So it is no surprise I failed the exam. |

| EFFORT:<br>internal, unstable, controllable | LUCK:<br>external, unstable, uncontrollable |
|---|---|
| e.g. I used subpar study strategies. Therefore, I will work harder next time and use up-to-date study strategies. | e.g. I was unlucky with the short answer questions they asked me. So I hope that they ask me questions I know next time. |

These attributions provide a framework for beliefs around failure and relate those beliefs to subsequent motivation in future efforts. Looking at these different attributions, you can explain this to yourself in four ways when you fail. How you explain this failure to yourself influences how you cope with failure and respond to future challenges to avoid failure.

Viewing failure as within your control has
profound implications for how you respond to failure
and the coping mechanisms that you use.

## LET'S UNPACK THIS IDEA A BIT MORE.

As shown in the table above, you can see ability is an internally perceived locus but out of the control of the individual. For example, the common perceived cause of failure is, *"I just can't pass these exams, and I never will."* In this case, the stable cause leads to low expectations for future success, while the internal and uncontrollable aspect leads to lower self-esteem. In addition, shame and humiliation are likely experienced. We can see this in Vignette 3, in which Salek doubts he can pass the exam and there is the subsequent stress and anxiety that follows.

Similarly, chance and luck are perceived as not having control but are external, unstable, and uncontrollable. *"I was unlucky that the wrong questions came up; maybe I'll be luckier next time,"* would be a general response if you fell into that bucket.

Another type of attribution that's common is, *"It's too difficult."* This is external, stable, and uncontrollable. For example, *"That's an impossible test, and it's no wonder I didn't pass."* These attributions are likely to lead to a sense of learned helplessness and a lack of hope.

A lack of effort is another commonly perceived cause of failure, and this is attributed as internal, unstable, and controllable. For example, *"I didn't study very smart; I could try harder next time."* Attribution to this factor maintains a sense of hope while at the same time eliciting guilt, which motivates you to amend the past. If you view your failure as a lack of effort, then you're likely to view past failures and future failures as in your control, and you'll use productive strategies to avoid a repeat scenario.

When failing, which is a stressor, one response could be to engage in problem-solving. Growth-minded doctors (such as Mohammed in Vignette 2 above) see a challenge as something they can overcome with effort. They are more likely to use adaptive coping strategies and respond better to failure.

One day, Kell took his four-year-old son to the park to play. Will was an extroverted child with great confidence and poise. He walked up to a new girl in the park and asked, *"Hey, do you want to play with me?"* The girl walked off without saying anything to him.

Kell was curious about how Will might take what could be construed as a rejection. When Will turned around, he said, *"Dad, that girl was shy – she doesn't talk,"* Kell was thinking, *"Wow, I hope that he brings that appraisal of the situation when he's at dating age."*

Now Will could have construed this rejection with an internal attribution – *"She doesn't like me,"* which tends towards the stable but uncontrollable attribution because there's not much Will can do about being a likeable person. This response to that rejection is more likely to have been damaging and had negative impacts on his self-esteem and self-worth than Will's actual response. This highlights that it is not what happens to us but rather the meaning we make of what happens to us that influences our emotions and reactions to the situation. And the good news is that we have the power to shift our thinking around this.

## ATTRIBUTION RETRAINING

There are two steps to consider in attribution retraining.

**1. Question your attribution.** Maladaptive attributions of failure that make doctors feel helpless are unhelpful. Ask yourself, *"What attributions am I making for failure or a setback?"* If you attribute failure to uncontrollable causes, such as those mentioned above, these are likely to be maladaptive attributions to failure.

**2. Devise an alternative**. If you notice that you're making a maladaptive attribution, can you devise alternative attributions? For example, instead of Mary saying, *"I failed because it was a difficult exam, and I can't pass these exams,"* she could replace this ability attribution with an effort attribution, *"I failed because I didn't use the study techniques in this textbook, I relied on re-reading the text."*

This attribution retraining helps you attribute the failure to a controllable cause that can be worked on for a better outcome in the future.

Attribution training might feel awkward, a little bit like crossing your arms the other way. Overcoming this discomfort comes through learning to suspend your disbelief. If you don't fully believe what you're trying to tell yourself, give yourself a score out of 10 and acknowledge that, no matter how little you believe this alternative, it is possible.

## DEALING WITH THOSE DIFFICULT FEELINGS

Failure is stressful, and how you cope with failure builds your resilience. In our experience, doctors who fail feel a gamut of emotions from shame and embarrassment or even worthlessness to anger and sadness. In Chapter Four, we talked briefly about the stress bucket, how stress increases the water in that bucket, and that there are taps that help reduce the stress and false taps that give short-term relief yet ultimately increase stress in the long run.

Doctors are at a higher risk of depression, anxiety, and burnout than the general population. This is because the nature of their work is highly demanding and stressful. Along with the long work hours and the competing priorities of work and personal lives, this can harm doctors' wellbeing. This is particularly true for junior doctors, according to the *National Mental Health Survey of Doctors and Medical Students* conducted by Beyond Blue.

Often, the junior doctors who visit us are dealing with failure in their exams. In our experience, their natural response is to avoid or suppress negative feelings that hurt. This can bring relief in the short term, but remember those false taps that we talked about in Chapter Four? Those maladaptive coping strategies can get in the way of processing emotion and can perpetuate those same feelings.

In addition to these negative emotions, many of our clients also feel self-critical after an exam failure. They can start to ruminate and overthink. If they're not careful, this can become a habit that perpetuates stress and burnout. To avoid this, they need to deal with those feelings using adaptive coping strategies.

Coping strategies can be adaptive or maladaptive.

- Adaptive coping strategies tend to involve identifying the stressor and using techniques that include confronting the problems directly or recognising the unhealthy emotions arising and healthily dealing with them.
- Maladaptive coping strategies might provide short-term relief, but overall do not address the underlying issues and contribute to stress in the long run.

The coping strategies that you chose can help you deal with the stress of being a junior doctor. According to a study of resilience, burnout, and coping mechanisms among UK doctors published in the *British Medical Journal*, maladaptive coping strategies, behavioural disengagement, substance abuse, and venting made significant contributions to the development of burnout.

## What you can do right now to make a change

### REVIEW YOUR COPING STRATEGIES

Coping strategies are context-dependent, so ultimately, you need to consider the context you are in. For example, taking a break from medicine for a year after failing your exam might be an adaptive coping strategy for someone who's a single parent of four young children and caring for their elderly parents. On the other hand, the same strategy might not be adaptive for someone who just needs to fine-tune their study skills. Context aside, here are several of the most common coping strategies doctors use in response to failure, setbacks, and stress. In the table, we have considered whether they would be adaptive or maladaptive. In the examples provided, we have provided doctors' authentic voices in response to the failure of their exams.

| COPING SKILL | DEFINITION | EXAMPLES FROM DOCTORS AFTER FAILING THEIR EXAM | ADAPTIVE OR MALADAPTIVE |
|---|---|---|---|
| Self-distraction | Focusing more explicitly on doing things to take one's mind off the stressor. | "I'm so stressed I can't study and am going to watch TV." | Maladaptive |
| Planning | Trying to come up with a strategy about what to do. | "I'm going to work out a study schedule and communicate this to my partner." | Adaptive |
| Emotional Support | Seeking emotional support from others. | "I am so stressed that I failed. Can I have a chat with you about it?" | Adaptive |
| Acceptance | Accepting and learning to live with the stressor. | "It's happened, and I can't change it, but I can learn from it and improve." | Adaptive |

| COPING SKILL | DEFINITION | EXAMPLES FROM DOCTORS AFTER FAILING THEIR EXAM | ADAPTIVE OR MALADAPTIVE |
|---|---|---|---|
| Rumination | Repeatedly replaying in your mind the stressful event and your role in it. | "I failed my exam. There is no way I will become a good doctor. I may as well leave the profession." | Maladaptive |
| Active coping | Focusing on doing something about the situation. | "I failed because I couldn't organise my time. I am going to enrol in a time-management course." | Adaptive |
| Self-blame | Criticising oneself for responsibility in the situation. | "I am so stupid and hopeless." | Maladaptive |
| Venting | Focussing on distress. | "I went home and vented with my wife about the exam." | Maladaptive |
| Instrumental support | Seeking help or advice from others on what to do. | "I have failed, and I am seeking help from a coach about how to manage my time and also study more effectively." | Adaptive |
| Behavioural disengagement | Giving up trying to cope or deal with the stressor. | "I don't know what to do or who to turn to. I am so upset I am not going to turn up to tutorials for the next little while." | Maladaptive |
| Denial | Trying to push the reality of the situation away. | "I refuse to believe that this has happened to me." | Maladaptive |

The specific coping strategies you use in response to exam failure or other setbacks can help you to solve your problems and support your wellbeing (adaptive coping). Alternatively, the coping strategies may provide temporary relief yet prevent the underlying issues or emotions from being resolved (maladaptive coping). Recognising that context matters, if you notice that you use a maladaptive coping strategy to deal with exam failure or other setbacks, then consider a more adaptive coping strategy in the table above.

## SUMMARY

Working as a doctor is a complex job in a highly dynamic environment where stressors exist from integrating disease presentation with diagnostic and treatment options to the politics and human factors in the work environment from both patients and colleagues. Trainee doctors need to respond well to those challenges and the inevitable failures that follow. Even though challenges and failure are confronting, having adaptive responses will enable you to succeed. In this chapter, we talked about three different factors:

- **Mindset.** A growth mindset means you're more likely to have more resilience, approach challenges, and respond better to criticism and failure than if you have a fixed mindset, which keeps you stuck. Here we provided the *yet* solution.

- **Attribution of failure**. Attributions influence your sense of self-worth and ability to bounce back. Being aware of how you attribute failure and then challenging yourself to try attribution is more likely to result in a better response to failure.

- **Adaptive coping skills.** Failure is painful, and it's easy to avoid these feelings and emotions. Here we looked at some adaptive coping skills that we often suggest to junior doctors with whom we work.

Considering the approach to failure in exam performance will reflect your coping strategies for your entire career – the job is a complex and dynamic one, even on a good day. Practising useful adaptive responses will contribute to your resilience and, therefore, capacity to succeed professionally.

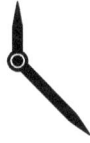

CHAPTER NINE

# SUCCESS IS ACHIEVABLE! BUT WHAT IS SUCCESS?

**R**eframe success. Bring success back to the elements you can control. It's more than exams. It's about your life – not burning out but having resilience and maintaining relationships and wellbeing. To succeed, you must manage failure. If you can learn this, you will become a better person. You can learn from your mistakes, which this book is all about. You can pass on these life and study skills to your kids and to young doctors who may work with you in the future instead of perpetuating that toxic medical system.

Most junior doctors have a narrow view of success. It's about passing exams. However, success can be defined in many ways. The Oxford Dictionary defines success as *"the attainment of object, wealth, fame, et cetera"*. We disagree with this definition. We define success as achieving a reasonable level of financial stability while doing work you enjoy and then finding that you are also happy and fulfilled with your life and career choices as well.

Yet not all doctors succeed at their final exam attempt or get invited to a specialty training program of their choosing. Some doctors choose or are forced to change their specialty. While we know that passing is what matters to you, we suggest you broaden your definition of success. Broadening your definition of success leads to a happier outcome overall and better mental health. It's long overdue to change the medical system. We've had inequities in society and the medical system for a long time.

Junior doctors suffer from fatigue due to insufficient breaks, long hours, and excessive overtime – often unpaid. This fatigue increases clinical errors, as we'll show you later in this chapter. The COVID pandemic has exacerbated this dysfunctional system. It revealed the extreme inequities for junior doctors and ancillary staff and has increased a lot of the overtime and the pressure. We've had Royal Commissions in other areas; maybe there needs to be one in the medical industry.

According to many comments in newspapers during the pandemic, when Australia needed our medical practitioners and nurses most, we treated them badly. Working excessive hours was exacerbated by the pandemic. There has been no improvement in bullying and intimidation of junior doctors, despite increased awareness.

We know that life after exams is essential too. Beyond passing the Fellowship exams, broadening your definition of success leads to a happier outcome overall and better mental health. Think about the reasons you've picked up this book in the first place. You may have been struggling with study and life balance. Most doctors suffer under an unfair system in silence. You dare not be a whistle-blower. It's easier to read this book than to complain. You start to think it's normal, but it's not! You've become acclimated to the toxic situation. When you get through those exams and start work as a consultant, you could be in a better position to do something about those inequities in the medical system. They will still be there long after you have passed your exams unless you join with others to help change the system.

Caroline Elton, an occupational psychologist in the United Kingdom, has been working with doctors for the last 20 years. In her 2018 book, *Also Human*, she examines why some doctors are overwhelmed by the pressures of medicine while others thrive. She describes, through case histories, the psychological and emotional problems that junior doctors can face. The case histories highlight the challenging pressures that many junior doctors deal with on a day-to-day basis. As Caroline Elton states, this occurs in the United Kingdom and here in Australia.

In November 2021, Lucy Carroll, the health reporter with the *Sydney Morning Herald*, reported the results of a hospital health check survey. This survey was undertaken with about 1,800 trainees during the peak of the New South Wales Delta COVID outbreak. It was conducted by the New South Wales Australian Medical Association and found that:

- almost 40% of junior doctors said they made a medical error due to the stress of working excessive hours
- 47% felt their personal safety was at risk from fatigue
- 60% worked more than five hours of unrostered overtime in an average fortnight during 2021 (compared to 50% in 2020)
- 723 junior doctors reported being bullied, mostly by senior medical officers
- 37% experienced intimidation – verbal or physical threats – from patients and/or families.

According to the survey, it *"reveals no major improvements in junior medicos being bullied and intimidated in the past five years..."* That's somewhat depressing, isn't it!

## REFRAME SUCCESS – FOCUS ON CONTROLLABLE ELEMENTS

Events may be beyond your control, but you entirely control your reactions to events. The first chapter of this book was about your reality as a junior doctor. The second, third, and fourth chapters were about wellbeing, resilience, and studying smarter. These included elements you can control, such as stress levels, studying smarter, and exercise. Your study becomes more efficient if you control those elements.

> Understanding that you have control over how you think, eat and exercise leads to greater resilience. Your sabotaging thoughts decrease, and your energy increases. You are more likely to remember what you study.

If you don't make changes, life will go on as before.

### MARIA'S STORY

*Maria had already had two attempts at her emergency medicine Fellowship exam and had failed both times. Both these attempts were during the first two years of COVID, and her exams were postponed and/or altered during that time. She worried that the dates for the next exams would be changed again and that the format could be changed as well. Maria was now 34 and was concerned about finding a partner. She felt that three of her girlfriends were doing better than her. They had passed the exams and were now either dating or engaged to be married.*

*Maria was starting to wonder if this was the right specialty for her. She was anxious, and her sabotaging thoughts led to a lack of motivation to study. She was eating lots of comfort food and was doing very little exercise. She was also exhausted because of the long working hours and extra overtime. It took an hour each day to drive to work at a major teaching hospital and another hour to drive home at the end of her shift.*

*Maria was upset about factors that were outside her control. She could foresee that her third attempt at the exam would be another failure unless she made some changes. This motivated her. She became more determined and focused. She ate healthily and sang her favourite songs in the car on her long drives to and from work. She even stopped at a beach on her way home from work to just walk and meditate. The effects were immediate. Maria's motivation to study and pass the exam increased. Her sabotaging thoughts decreased. Some weeks later, we received an email – she had finally passed. "Thank you SO much for your words of wisdom and for helping me prepare a game plan – it made a huge difference! And I will be taking the lessons learned forward."*

## What you can do right now to make a change

### START A TRAINING DIARY

It's a good idea to keep a training diary allocated for all the activities you do daily that will help you pass the upcoming exams. Include all the activities you did that day to increase wellbeing and mental health and also record the quality of any study or testing. We would suggest a week-to-view diary as you can then keep tabs on your activities over a week. Always keep a score, with ten being excellent, and zero being poor or not done that day. For example, on wellbeing, you might be thinking about increasing your exercise. It's good for your overall health, and you will be able to focus more readily. You decide to increase your walking and maybe go for a jog once or twice a week. At the end of each day, you open your diary and ask yourself this question. "Am I pleased with the exercise I did today?" If you are, give yourself a high score out of 10.

Or you may have read some research that indicated that excess sugar could impair memory in the brain cells. You are aware that you usually have three cups of coffee a day, with a heaped teaspoon of sugar in each cup. You decide to cut down on the amount of sugar in your coffee. At the end of the day, you write in your diary the question, "Am I pleased with the amount of sugar I cut down on today?" and give yourself an appropriate score out of 10.

Note the way the question has been worded. You are not berating yourself for not doing something adequately every day of the week. With shift work, family issues, overtime, etc., your scores could be different every day. Learn to be kind to yourself. Don't expect perfection.

The benefits are that the act of recording scores daily in your diary is likely to increase your motivation and your wellbeing. Once you have completed a week or two in your diary, look back and note your earlier scores. The act of evaluating yourself maintains your awareness of looking after your wellbeing. You are more likely to keep going. We use wellbeing as an example because it is more likely that you will be tempted to ignore it. In our experience, most doctors think focusing on wellbeing probably takes up too much of their precious study time.

## SUCCESS IS MORE THAN PASSING EXAMS

Success can also mean that you've learned to take charge of your emotions and behaviours – your fear of failure, your catastrophising, and even that imposter syndrome, which is more common than you think. You now have an increased awareness of your thoughts and feelings. You pause and take a breath before you react. Your actions are now more considered and thoughtful. You have reduced the chances of a less than optimal response.

Perhaps you have decided to insert a mindfulness exercise into your daily schedule. This leads to a sense of calm and a feeling of control. This calmness impacts your interactions positively with work colleagues and with family.

Learning to take charge of your emotions
and behaviours leads to better personal and
professional relationships throughout your life.
This is a measure of success.

## JOSIE'S STORY

*One of our clients, Josie, nearly walked away from medicine. She was
an accredited surgical program trainee and was continually bullied and
intimidated by a particular male consultant. This usually happened in
theatre when she was trying to focus while working on an anaesthetised
patient. (And this occurs more often than you might think! Imagine
being the patient!)*

*This poor doctor was terrified that she would make a mistake, but she
was also too scared to tell the consultant not to ask questions while she
was busy with the patient. She knew it would be held against her! On
one occasion, Josie politely asked him to stop questioning her until after
the surgery. He just shrugged his shoulders and said, "You're a woman;
you can multitask."*

*However, after lots of practice, Josie learned to take a diaphragmatic
breath after the consultant's question. This pause enabled her to take
more control of when she would answer the question. She felt less worried
about making mistakes, and she was able to switch focus, briefly answer
the consultant, and return to her patient. This, for her, was an essential
measure of success.*

We want to see more female consultant surgeons. Any step in that direction
is a measure of success. Currently, only 12% of surgeons in Australia are
women. We'd like that to increase.

Here is a fun exercise we do with junior doctors. They soon get the point.
We get them to turn on the audio recording on their phone. Then one of
us asks, *"Please give me your name, your occupation, and your hospital."* There is

usually an *"um"* or some other word such as *"okay"* before giving the name. They usually stutter a little over the occupation and hospital, and they forget what we asked.

What is happening is that these doctors, like most of us, tend to blurt out an answer without thinking because they don't like the silence. They don't get the initial words of the sentence sorted out before they start speaking, so they sound hesitant. We have all done this.

Then we ask them the same question again after turning on the recording device, but they must take a big breath before they commence their answer. Usually, this time the doctor takes a big breath in but can't wait and starts their answer before they complete the breath. We laugh about it and try again and again. Eventually, it works, and what a difference! The voice is clear and concise, the words are deliberate with no word fillers. They now have all the answers recorded on their phone and can, at their leisure, listen to the improvement on each repetition.

Finally, we get our client to ask the same question of one of us. We make sure we pause and breathe in and out before answering. When we later ask, *"Was that pause too long?"*, the answer is *"No, you appeared thoughtful, as though you were considering your response."* We tell them that that is exactly how they seemed when they took a big breath before answering. This is reassuring for them. In most cases, they felt that they were pausing too long before answering.

Being able to pause and focus before answering
questions under pressure is also a measure of success.

## BARRIERS TO SUCCESS – THE HOSPITAL SYSTEM IN AUSTRALIA

We have given you a lot of advice on what you can do in your exams. But the reality is that you are in a dysfunctional system. We are not blaming you for these systemic problems. We're helping you to cope. As authors and psychologists, we would love this system to change. We would like to see more compassion and awareness of psychological and physical issues that cause junior doctors to fail. We would like to see changes in the system – and we would love you to be involved in these changes down the track. We're talking about when you are a consultant and have young doctors under your care, and when you are respected and liked for the way you help train these junior doctors. Given the opportunity, later, we'd love to see you join committees or working groups that are involved with the welfare of young doctors. It's not your fault that you are physically and psychologically exhausted by your job and maintaining a life outside work. There is only so much you can do when you are working around the clock. But when you are a consultant, you could make a difference.

Amanda Howe and her colleagues wrote an interesting article in 2012, "Towards an Understanding of Resilience and its Relevance to Medical Training". They stated that doctors must be resilient if they are to survive the long, gruelling training and the constant exposure to death, distress, and disability that medicine brings. They need to be adaptable and flexible – able to absorb the pressures of work, the stresses of medicine, and the ethical and moral challenges associated with being a modern doctor.

In a more recent 2015 article, "Doctors Need to be Supported, Not Trained in Resilience", Eleanor Balme and colleagues went further. They pointed out that resilience is a complex and dynamic interplay between the individual, the individual's environment, and sociocultural factors. Interventions to promote resilience must deal with organisational as well as individual and team issues. Here is a small part of a five-page letter that Kell's 30-year-old ambitious self wrote:

*"Dear future me, today is your 45th birthday. Take a breath and look upwards and outwards. Do you feel the sunshine on your skin? Are you grateful for the opportunities that have come your way? In the past, you have often gravitated to*

*work. So, make sure you take a moment and step outside, away from the pressures of work and deadlines, without feeling guilty. Take some time out for yourself and smell the flowers..."*

Kell looked at it again when he was 45, with three children and a successful teaching career. However, when he looked over the letter, he realised how he turned out differently from his expectations of himself – how life turned out differently and how fast time flies. Advice and wisdom are conventionally passed from elders to youth, parents to children, and the experienced to the novice. He found that writing a letter to his future self was an exercise in compassion, self-love, and a reminder of what is most important to an older, more worn version of himself.

He was reminded of what was most important and the value of doing favours for his future self, such as taking time out to have a healthy mind and body, cultivating loving and meaningful relationships, providing lots of great memories, and that he works to live and not lives to work.

Perhaps you could write a letter to your future self as Kell did. There are several things to consider when writing this letter. These can be segmented into a few different areas. Set the tone by asking questions.

1. What lessons have I learned up until this point in life?
2. What goals have I achieved? Who has helped me, and how did I thank them?
3. Am I happy, and what are the things that make me happy?
4. What is important to me? Am I spending enough time on the things that matter to me? Do I spend enough time looking after my health and wellbeing?
5. Am I living according to my expectations or what others expect of me?

What are your current beliefs that you want to share with your future self? Share your beliefs in the different areas of life that resonate for you (family, friends, health, relationships, money, career, spirituality).

What do you want to change in the future? This vital part of the letter creates a bridge between your current self and a better version of yourself.

1. What should I remember?
2. What goals do I have for the future?
3. What meaningful relationships need more attention, and do I need to reconsider some relationships?
4. What things should I add or exclude from my life?
5. What habits and practices could I do to be healthier?

You can use this software to write a letter to your future self which then sends it to your email in the future: https://www.futureme.org/

## SUMMARY

Success, like a diamond, has many facets. Yes, you want to pass your exams, but you also want to be able to communicate under pressure. You want to look and feel confident. You want to tame those sabotaging thoughts. You can use the skills you have learned in this book now and in the future. Perhaps you need to change your mindset. The difference between an ordeal and a challenge is attitude. You can be successful in so many ways.

Focus on using your new skills. First, use them in familiar surroundings. As you become more skilled, use them in intimidating scenarios. Clarity comes with action.

# CONCLUSION

## WHAT HAVE I LEARNED?

You can ace your medical exams AND have a wonderful life prioritising your family, friends, health, and wellbeing. You have learned how you can survive a toxic medical system that doesn't always look after the psychological and physical wellbeing of its trainees. You didn't know what you were signing up for in med school. You didn't realise how hard you had to study in the ten or more years after graduation, that you would still be doing exams, or how it would impact other areas of your life. You've read this book. Give it a go. You are not going to get it right all the time. The system is dysfunctional, and it often works against you. But you now have some psychological techniques that work.

There is a huge gap between the advances made in medical practice and our understanding of the psychological impact of medical work. The technological advances are amazing, but the way trainees and other healthcare workers must put up with various stressors hasn't changed over the decades. As medical students and junior doctors, you are taught about patient-centred care. You are taught how to communicate with patients and show empathy to their needs – it's drummed into you from day one. But what about care towards you, the junior doctors? You're stressed – physically, emotionally, and mentally. The exhaustion, the responsibility, and the fear of making mistakes can weigh heavily.

You know that by practising the psychological and non-verbal techniques you have just read about; you will look and feel more confident when consultants fire questions at you. You can imagine stepping up and being the first to answer questions on clinical rounds. You must answer these types of questions in exams, so why not now? What have you got to lose? So what if you fear giving a wrong answer and feel you are making a fool of yourself? It's only those sabotaging thoughts that hold you back from demonstrating your newfound courage to speak up. You can also show that same courage at home. When you need help, ask for it. You don't get medals for being a martyr.

Just because you've read about these psychological techniques and done them once or twice, that doesn't mean you'll always do them successfully under pressure.

Deliberate, repeated practice of every single technique you choose to do will pay dividends. You'll soon see – life will be so much better.

However, there may be continuing uncertainty and adverse effects that could derail your work and study. The COVID pandemic is a fantastic example. There may be well-meaning consultants and fellows who advise you to study 12 hours a day on your days off. There will be other consultants who are intimidating and resist your attempts to change. Wouldn't you prefer to stick to scientific principles and decades of collective experience from the two of us rather than anecdotal advice?

In this book, you've learned how to deal with negative thoughts, look after your body and mind, and study and test to suit the mature brain. You may have your doubts at times; the advice in this book probably contradicts everything you have ever heard about passing exams and your own experience. But we can say without hesitation that this works because it is based on science and our experience.

You may fall by the wayside occasionally, but that is just being human. Pick yourself up and persist. Soon, good habits will replace bad habits. Taking control of your actions will lead to success in your personal and professional life – both before and after those pesky exams.

To make real and lasting change, you must be persistent. Now that you've read the book, this is the beginning of a new you.

Start small. Don't do every technique at once.
At first, try one or two that attract you
and fit into your lifestyle.

Do lots of repetition. This is how new habits are formed, and old habits die for good. You can look forward to increased success in many areas of your life. In this book, you have everything you need to succeed. But if you'd like more help applying these principles to your life, that is what we do. We coach doctors who want guidance on how to ace their medical exams.

We long for a time when it isn't necessary to write how-to care-for-yourself books for junior doctors. We want the medical profession to consciously consider medical service's psychological and physical impacts on trainees and make positive changes. Our wish for the future is to see the medical colleges and the hospital administrations throughout Australia take more steps to care for medical trainees' wellbeing. Doctors have a challenging journey from the early years in medical school to finally becoming consultants.

We need to take care of our medics. After all, they take care of us. But until that golden day, this book has given you the power to take care of yourself.

.

# ACKNOWLEDGEMENTS

We made it! Late nights, early mornings, trying to squeeze some writing in during little breaks during the day. Collaborating with each other via Zoom and phone calls when we needed it. We learned a lot along the way. It's a little bit like running a 10K race – torture in the middle, but then you look back on it and think "well, that wasn't so bad".

However, we had lots of help and guidance. First, we'd like to thank Kath Walters, our editor and book coach. She was so insightful with her comments, guiding us through the book planning, and the writing of the first draft, always keeping us on our toes. We couldn't have asked for a better coach, as Kath combined kindness and supportiveness with exceptional editorial skills when we started flagging and getting behind.

Then the first draft was finished, and it went out to our first readers – mostly consultants, fellows, and senior registrars in various specialties. They gave so very generously of their time, especially when hospitals around the country have been so short-staffed. The feedback was so valuable from these experts in the field and helped to inform our understanding of the psychological demands of medical work. We have not shared their names, but these doctors were extraordinarily helpful with their incisive comments. However, there is one person, Colin Jones, to whom we can give a shout-out. He is not a medic but has been involved for many years in the airline and IT industries. Colin was able to give a fresh non-medical perspective and some interesting and different suggestions.

We have drawn on the stories and anecdotes from a range of clients over the years. A big thank you to them. They have shared their failures, their fears, their hopes, their successes, and their dreams. And where appropriate we have shared their stories with our readers. Their names and identifying details have, of course, been changed to protect their identity.

We are very grateful to the doctors who have taken the time to write testimonials about the book, and to Professor Mohamed Khadra, who again has provided a terrific foreword.

Thank you, also, to Lu Sexton, Wordsmith. It was amazing what Lu could do to tidy up our writing. She cut out the material or placed it elsewhere. She knew what worked! We are both academics, and we think we're used to writing clear and concise research grants – weren't we in for a surprise!

Then off to the proofreader, Stephanie Preston. By this time, we had no illusions about our writing – we knew there would be lots of little things that had been overlooked and that Stephanie would find them. We accidentally discovered that one other person with a keen eye for finding proofing errors was Cy, a family member.

We searched through photos and just couldn't find any of the two of us together, for the book cover, so went to an expert, Sharon Hickey, for some photos. Finding a day when we were both free was somewhat of a challenge.

Then eventually, heaving a sigh of relief, the book was in the final stages. Our book designer, the very creative Liz Seymour, from Seymour Designs, had waited patiently for us to finish. We had juggled the dates to get the book to her on several occasions. Liz had designed the first book, *Ace Your Medical Exams*, so we were grateful that she was available to design this second book.

And finally, a big thank you to our family and friends. They were supportive in so many ways. Whether it was through the provision of encouragement or technical support, late-night conversations around the dining room table, or taking care of the kids when deadlines were approaching. They were encouraging when it all felt too difficult. We are grateful for the love and support that our family and friends have given us. This book is for them, and for all the up-and-coming junior doctors who are on that gruelling journey to become consultants.

# BIBLIOGRAPHY

Adderholdt, Miriam, Johnson, Donna, & Levy, Nathan. (2016). *Perfectionism vs. The Pursuit of Excellence: What Can be Bad About Being Too Good*. USA: Nathan Levy Books.

Allen, David. (2003). *Ready for Anything: 52 Productivity Principles for Work and Life*. USA: Penguin Books.

AMA *Position Statement on the Health and Wellbeing of Doctors and Medical Students 2020* is available at https://ama.com.au/position-statement/health-and-wellbeing-doctors-andmedical-students-2020

Balme, Eleanor, et al. (2015). *Doctors Need to be Supported, not Trained in Resilience*. BMJ Publishing Group.

Beyond Blue. (2013). *National Mental Health Survey of Doctors and Medical Students*. Australia: Beyond Blue.

Blackwell, Lisa, Trzesniewski, Kali, & Dweck, Carol. (2007). Implicit Theories of Intelligence Predict Achievement Across Adolescent Transition: A Longitudinal Study and an Intervention. *Child Development*. USA: Blackwell Publishing.

Blomstrand, Peter & Engvall, Jan. (2021). Effects of a Single Exercise Workout on Memory and Learning Functions in Young Adults – A Systematic Review. *Translational Sports Medicine*. Open Access: Wiley.

McKinley, Nicola et al. (2019). Resilience, Burnout, and Coping Mechanisms in UK Doctors: A Cross-Sectional Study. *British Medical Journal* Open 2020;10: e031765. doi:10.1136.

Carney, Dana; Cuddy, Amy; & Yap, Andy. (2010). Power Posing: Brief Nonverbal Displays Affect Neuroendocrine Levels and Risk Tolerance. *Psychological Science*, Oct. 21, (10),1363–8.

Carroll, Lucy. (2021). NSW Australian Medical Association Hospital Health Check Survey. *Sydney Morning Herald*, Nov.

Clark, Roy, Peter. (2013). *How to Write Short: Word Craft for Fast Times*. USA: Little, Brown Spark.

Clear, James (2018) *Atomic Habits: An Easy & Proven Way to Build Good Habits and Break Bad Ones*. UK: Random House.

Dunlosky, John, et al. (2013). Improving Student's Learning with Effective Learning Techniques: Promising Directions From Cognitive and Educational Psychology. *Psychological Science in the Public Interest*.

Dwek, Carol. (2007). *Mindset: The New Psychology of Success*. USA: Ballantine Books.

Ebersbach, Mirjam, & Nazari, Katherine. (2020). Implementing Distributed Practice in Statistics Courses: Benefits for Retention and Transfer. *Journal of Applied Research in Memory and Cognition*, 9, (4), 532–541.

Ebbinghaus, Hermann. (1913). Memory: A Contribution to Experimental Psychology. Annals of Neurosciences. 20, (4) Oct.

Elton, Caroline. (2018). *Also Human: The Inner Lives of Doctors*. UK: Penguin Random House.

Encyclopedia Britannica, www.britannica.com/

Epstein, David. (2019). *Range: Why Generalists Triumph in a Specialized World*. USA: Riverhead Books.

Ferris, Timothy. (2011). *The 4-Hour Workweek*. UK: Vermillion, A Random House Group.

Frankl, Viktor (1946). *Man's Search for Meaning*. USA: Beacon Press.

Gladwell, Malcolm. (2005). *Blink: The Power of Thinking without Thinking*. USA: Little, Brown, and Co.

Gladwell, Malcolm. (2008). *Outliers: The Story of Success*. USA: Little, Brown, and Co.

Glass, Arnold & Kang, Mengxue. (2020). Fewer Students are Benefiting from Doing their Homework: An Eleven-year Study. *Educational Psychology*. Published online.

Goldin, Sarah, (1979). Recognition Memory for Chess Positions. Some Preliminary Research. *The American Journal of Psychology*, 92, (1), 19–31.

Hoffman, et al. (2010). The Effect of Mindfulness-based Therapy on Anxiety and Depression: A Meta-analytic Review. *Journal of Consulting and Clinical Psychology, 78,* (2),169.

Holmes, Paul, & Collins, David. (2001). The PETTLEP Approach to Mental Imagery: A Functional Equivalence Model for Sport Psychologists. *Journal of Applied Sport Psychology, 13,* (1), 60–83.

Howe, Amanda, et al. (2012). Towards an Understanding of Resilience and its Relevance to Medical Training. *Medical education*, 46, (4),349–356.

Jandial, Rahul. (2019). *Life Lessons from a Brain Surgeon*. UK.: Penguin Random House.

Jones, E.E., Kanouse, D.E., Kelley, H.H., Nisbett, R.E., Valins, S., & Weiner, B., (Eds.), (1976). *Attribution: Perceiving the Causes of Behavior*. USA: Lawrence Erlbaum Associates, Inc,

Jordan, Michael, National Basketball Association. star in Nike Ad, 1997.

Kabat-Zinn, Jon. (2016). *Mindfulness for Beginners: Reclaiming the Present Moment – And your Life*. USA: Sounds True Inc.

Kahneman, Daniel. (2011), *Thinking, Fast and Slow*. UK: Penguin Books.

Karpicke, J. & Blunt, J. (2011) Retrieval Practice Produces More Learning than Elaborative Studying with Concept Mapping. *Science*, 331, (6018),772–775.

Manson, Mark. (2016). *The Subtle Art of Not Giving a F\*CK: A Counterintuitive Approach to Living a Good Life*. USA: Harper-Collins.

Mether, Leah. (2019). *Soft is the New Hard*. Australia: Methmac Communications.

Moors, Agnes, & De Houwer, Jan. (2006). Automaticity: A Theoretical and Conceptual Analysis. *The Psychological Bulletin*, 132, (2),297.

Murre, Jaap, & Dros, Joeri. (2015). Replication and Analysis of Ebbinghaus' Forgetting Curve. *Computer Science*, PLoS ONE 10, (7).

Navarro, J. (2008). *What Everybody Is Saying: An Ex-FBI Agent's Guide to Speed-reading People*. USA: Harper-Collins.

Ratey, John, J. (2013). *Spark: The Revolutionary New Science of Exercise and the Brain*. USA: Little, Brown Spark.

Roediger, Henry, & Karpicke, Jeffrey. (2006). Test-enhanced Learning: Taking Memory Tests Improves Long-term Retention. *Psychological Science*, 17, (3), 249–255.

Routh, Zoe. (2020). *People Stuff: Beyond Personality Problems*. Australia: Inner Compass.

Sheehan, Martina, & Pearse, Susan. (2017). *Do Less and Be More: Ban Busy and Make Space for What Matters*. Australia: Hay House.

Smith, Huston. (1999). *The World's Religions: Our Great Wisdom Traditions*. San Francisco: Harper.

Smith, Kristopher & Apicella, Coren. (2017). Winners, Losers and Posers: The effect of Power Poses on Testosterone and Risk-taking Following Competition. *Hormones and Behavior*. UK: Elsevier.

Tawfik, Daniel;Profit, Jochen; Webber, Sarah; & Tait, Shanafelt. (2019). Organizational Factors Affecting Physician Well-being. *Current Treatment Options in Pediatrics*, 5, 11–25.

Tremayne, Patsy. (2019). *Ace Your Medical Exams*, Australia: Ingram Spark.

Vealey, Robin., & Greenleaf, Christy.. (2006). Seeing is Believing: Understanding and Using Imagery in Sport. In Jean M. Williams (Ed.), *Applied Sport Psychology: Personal Growth to Peak Performance. (5th ed.,)*. USA: McGraw Hill.

Walters, Kath. (2020). *Overnight Authority*. Australia: Sticky Content.

Weiner, B., Frieze, I., Kukla, A., Reed, L., Rest, S., & Rosenbaum, R. M. (1987). Perceiving the causes of success and failure. In *Preparation of this paper grew out of a workshop on attribution theory held at University of California, Los Angeles, Aug 1969.*. USA: Lawrence Erlbaum Associates, Inc..

Westbrook, J.I., Woods, A., Rob, M.I., Dunsmuir, W.T. & Day, R.O. (2010). Association of Interruptions with an Increased Risk and Severity of Medication Administration Errors. *Archives of Internal Medicine*, 170, (8), 683–690.

Williams, Jean (Ed). (2010). *Applied Sport Psychology: Personal Growth to Peak Performance*. USA: Mayfield Publishing Co.

World Health Organization. (2005). *Constitution of the World Health Organization*. World Health Organization: Basic documents. 45th ed. Geneva.

Yongzhi, Wang cited from Sun Tung-Tien. (2020). Active Versus Passive Reading: How to Read Scientific Papers. *National Science Review*, 7, (9). https://academic.oup.com/nsr/article/7/9/1422/5859953